New York Times Best-Selling Author of *Body by God*

WINNING

THE INSIDE
BATTLE OF

WELLNESS

OVERCOMING THE

MENTAL HURDLES

AND LIFE CHALLENGES

THAT STOP YOU FROM

STICKING TO A DIET

OR EXERCISE PLAN

DR. BEN LERNER

Winning the Inside Battle of Wellness: Overcoming the Mental Hurdles and Life Challenges That Stop You From Sticking to a Diet or Exercise Plan

by Dr. Ben Lerner

copyright ©2017 Dr. Ben Lerner

Trade paperback ISBN: 978-1-943294-55-8
Ebook ISBN: 978-1-943294-56-5

Winning the Inside Battle is also available on Amazon Kindle, Barnes & Noble Nook and Apple iBooks.

CONTENTS

1. EVERYONE'S BATTLE 5

2. BRAINWORKS 11

3. A BEAUTIFUL MIND 39

4. WINNING THE INSIDE BATTLE 69

5. "THE BAD LIFESTYLE" PSA 87

6. 10 TRICKS FOR A CHANGE 109

7. BREAKFAST AND SMOOTHIE RECIPES 175

8. LUNCH RECIPES 197

9. DINNER RECIPES 219

10. SNACK AND DESSERT RECIPES 243

ENDNOTES 261

chapter 1

EVERYONE'S BATTLE

MY EARLIEST MEMORY OF CHILDHOOD is a hospital. I can't remember my first dog being brought home as a puppy. I can't recall my first ice cream cone or scraped knee. But I can remember standing by the hospital bed of a very sick relative who was about to die. What a creepy, scary, dark place that hospital was. I believe that's the reason the memory is there. Some of the names, details, and faces are cloudy, but something one of the adults said to me that day is still crystal clear to me now. Looking right at me, she said: "This is how all of the people in your family end up at an early age."

I was either two or three years old at the time. That makes her either cruel or crazy! You'd have to be serial-killer cruel to say that to a toddler, so I'm guessing "crazy." Unable to judge emotional intelligence, IQ, or mental soundness at the time, I took the statement at face value. I thought: *I'll be dead soon.*

Thus, from the age of two or three, I became interested in health, lifestyle, and beating the odds of dying young while lying in some unhappy hospital bed.

This is no mere phobia, mind you. I am named after my grandfather, whom I never met. By the time I was a teenager, all four grandparents and my favorite uncle were gone. The expedient manner by which the members of my family left the planet caused me to pay attention to my parents' battle with their bodies with *grave* concern (pun intended).

OUR BATTLE

Mom and Dad both smoked. Dad smoked Camel cigarettes, no-filters. The Camel tagline in the 1970s was, "Where a Man Belongs." The ad campaign featured a brawny, mustached man doing manly outdoor things while smoking his Camel. My mom was a Marlboro woman, and the saying, "Light the next cigarette from the last one," was actually coined by someone who was watching them chain-smoke! In other words, they didn't need a lighter; they just lit their next cigarette from the burning end of the one they were smoking.

Perhaps the best illustration of their chain-smoking was our trips from Cleveland, Ohio, to White Plains, New York, to visit our cousins. Mom and Dad would pack my two brothers and I in the back seat of the Gremlin, seal the windows, and smoke for twelve straight hours. It was so smoky in that car, I had no idea how my dad could see out the windows to drive. The really rough moments were the burning eyes, the runny nose, the bleeding gums, and the yellowing that would form around our fingernails. On a positive note, at some point we kids all would pass out from tar and nicotine poisoning for the last seven to eight hours of the trip. This helped us avoid boredom and kill time before iPhones and in-car DVDs were invented. So we had that going for us!

For my parents, none of the smoking risks were mitigated by any action or inaction that could be considered remotely beneficial to their physical health. They did not exercise; they both really struggled with their weight, particularly my dad; food choices were unhealthy; and there were not any kinds of spiritual or religious practices present that could smooth out the rough emotional patches or calm any storms.

That was our battle. Many, many people face a similar battle or, of course, battle things much worse. My entire childhood was engrossed in this fight. I never stopped worrying about my parents, to the degree that I'm certain I probably drove them nuts and only made matters worse. I vowed to figure out one day how to help them, my brothers, and the millions like you who are in the battle as well.

Since the time I was two or three years old, I've wanted to make people's lives easier, not harder, to live than they are right now.

NATURE, NURTURE—OR NEITHER

When my dad was fifty-two, he died of a heart attack the night before we were leaving on a family vacation. My mom, who was still in her forties, became permanently disabled by a stroke a year later. It is accurate to say my dad lifestyled himself to death and that my mom's disability was self-induced.

As I write this, I am fifty. My cholesterol level is approximately half and my blood pressure is one-third less than what my dad's was. I am his same height and 25 percent lighter. Other than exposure to secondhand smoke as a child, I have avoided stepping on the many bad-lifestyle landmines that are buried in my genetic up-line.

When it comes to addiction, eating disorders, attitudes, personalities, obesity—any lifestyle or health problem—arguments exist over the causes. Some scientists believe the core cause is *nature*; others believe it is *nurture*. Meaning, is the cause rooted in genetics, or is it the way we are raised that screws us up?

Yet, in the case of my brothers and me, we each have the nature and an overwhelming amount of the nurture—but without the problematic outcomes of obesity, stress, musculoskeletal issues, and cardiovascular disease found in our patriarchs and matriarchs. And there is good reason for this difference. As science has evolved, we have come to realize that it is neither genes nor upbringing that makes the difference. It's choice. You don't have to win a battle of evolution to be healthy. You have to make better choices.

The solution is winning the *inside battle* of wellness.

The battle is a mental one; the unhealthy outcomes are not something we can really blame on our great-grandparents. The fact that you are struggling with your lifestyle is not an insult to your intelligence. My parents both were exceedingly book-smart. My mother earned a perfect score on her English SATs, which is ridiculous. No one does that. For my dad, an error in putting the CPA exam together for the state of New York when Dad sat for it caused everyone but three of the people taking it to fail. My dad was one of those three.

On the other hand, my dad would often say, "I'd rather be dead than eat this way." when he was on a diet. My mom, from my vantage point, frankly did not seem to give a darn about her body, based on what she'd eat, drink, and breathe. For her, like for many people, even having the stroke didn't stop her from smoking or improve the way she took care of her body.

When my dad said he'd rather die, or when my mom lived in a way that was akin to committing suicide, it does not mean they actually wanted to kill themselves. My dad loved us. What's more, he lived for us. He did not want to leave behind three kids and the wife he loved. My mom, the English genius, did not want to have a stroke that would result in her having trouble even understanding English the rest of her life. They were very smart people. But they lost the inside battle.

THERE IS AN ANSWER

I had the distinct worry, stress, and fear of watching every step of their journey for more than twenty years. They really struggled. When my dad said he'd "rather die," I completely understood. His knowledge of "healthy" at the time was eating "rabbit food" and taking long, boring walks on a treadmill. Their struggles, and the stress and fear it caused me, pushed me into more than thirty years of study. I completed a nutrition degree, became a chiropractor, and am working on a Ph.D. in psychology. I became an Advanced Personal Trainer and even taught the course. I've consulted for over 2,000 doctors, worked with over 1 million patients, and have written eighteen books, all to get the answers I didn't have for my dad and mom to others.

Looking back at the work I've put in, I'd say, yes, I've been pretty obsessed with finding solutions and creating tools to make living well easier. No one wants to live the "rabbit food" life my dad hated. The gospel truth and the good news of health is this: *you don't have to!*

My dad lost more than 1,000 pounds during his life but died weighing the same amount he weighed when he'd start one of his diets. Being healthy was just too hard for him— he lacked the knowledge, tools, and steps needed to make a good lifestyle doable long-term. I want you to understand that you don't have to panic and think, *I stink at the inside battle and I'll never get any better!* You will get better. Like my dad, you may simply lack the tools and steps you need to make your change possible. So take a deep breath, relax, and keep reading. On the pages that follow I'm going to give you the resources you need to win your inside battle.

chapter 2

BRAINWORKS

THE AREA OF OUR BRAINS that's responsible for executive functions is called the prefrontal cortex. Just as the president of the United States makes executive decisions from the Oval Office that affect the entire country, so activity in the prefrontal cortex our brain controls your body's policies on lifestyle affairs. The brain is like the body's Oval Office!

The prefrontal cortex is responsible for controlling consumption habits. A Canadian study at the University of Waterloo found that overeating junk food can be caused by errors in how this part of the brain functions.[1] The researchers, who published their findings in *Psychosomatic Medicine: Journal of Biobehavioral Medicine*, discovered that there were operational flaws in the prefrontal cortex in people who craved and ate the most junk food during the experiment.

This means that for some of us, the brain is working against us instead of for us. Thanks, brain!

Studies have also found that the brain's prefrontal areas can be an issue for people who struggle to control their behaviors. When high functioning, this part of the brain can manage automatic, knee-jerk type reactions like cravings for cheesecake, bread, or vodka and instead make better, healthier, long-term decisions on behalf of the body. When this part of the brain lapses or is "taken offline," cravings, bad snacking decisions, and overeating are boosted and rage against the machine.

Your brain provides the underlying circuitry that causes you to behave in certain ways. Utilizing technology, scientists can now see the location and action of brain activation related to what you are thinking. For example, if you view a picture of your family, your brain activity can be assessed. The occipital lobe of the brain will exhibit and increase in blood flow that is detectable on a functional MRI scan or seen as electrical activity on an EEG. Visual perception received in that part of the brain causes it to "fire."

Neuroscientists J. T. Kaplan, S. I. Gimbel, and S. Harris at the Brain and Creativity Institute at the University of Southern California studied another important area of the brain when it comes to your life's commitments. They found that when political beliefs are challenged, a person's brain becomes active in areas that govern personal identity and emotional responses to threats.[2] Those resistant to changing their beliefs had more activity in the amygdala—a pair of almond-shaped areas near the center of the brain and the insular cortex—compared with people who were more willing to change their minds. This study also revealed that abilities such as self-control and power to change and grow can be wired into our neural circuits.

The brain, its intricate neural connections, and its incredibly complex patterns of firing greatly influence perceptions and behaviors. Yet, you also possess "cognition," or the ability to think, evaluate ideas, process information, reflect, and become aware of the subtle beauty of life. The great news is you can change and improve both your brain and your thoughts. As you'll see in the next chapter, your brain, thoughts, and actions are not permanently preprogrammed. As both brain and cognition improve, you can move toward a true, metamorphic, caterpillar-to-butterfly-like change.

NEUROPLASTICITY

If you have a president in your body's Oval Office who's making bad decisions every day, don't worry. You're not stuck with him forever. The important parts of the brain like the prefrontal cortex and the amygdala can be built up, reconditioned, and remodeled, allowing you to better break free from neurologically induced habits.

Rebuilding and Remolding The Brain

Over the last several years, one of the most encouraging findings we have discovered about our future is that the brain can build, re-build, mold, and remold in order to better thrive and respond to its environment. This is called "neuroplasticity."

Think of plastic as something you can add to and mold and you'll better understand the concept of neuroplasticity. It allows the nervous system to rise above and go beyond any genetic limitations, current challenges, past experiences, or constraints and make the adaptations necessary to create a better future.

At one time, scientists thought that the brain's growing, molding, and adaptation process occurred in-womb only.

Now, thanks to one of the more exciting developments in recent biological history, we know the brain develops over the course of your entire life. The process of neuroplasticity occurs through the growth of new brain neurons and synaptogenesis—the growth of new nerve connections.

Your nervous system is always learning and making the necessary adaptations to excel in your environment, occupation, and overall mental and physical challenges. New neuron development, for example, occurs at an estimated rate of 2,000 per hour in the adult hippocampus. You have a new brain emerging every day, so never feel stranded with your old one! Your brain grows new nerve cells, molds them, and organizes and reorganizes them based on the input the brain is getting so that you can survive and thrive in your most common circumstances.

Making Your Brain Work For You Not Against you

Millions of people make New Year's resolutions every December 31. The preponderance of those resolutions are for getting into better shape. Sadly, nearly all of them fail to even get off the dock, and those that do mostly go down in the harbor—by about January 4! Lately I have noticed a trend: people just do not make resolutions anymore. The term *resolution* actually means "fixed purpose." In an effort to avoid kicking off the New Year with a failure by committing to a purpose that is anything but fixed, people have opted out of making one at all. I can't blame them. Who wants to set themselves up to fail?

You may believe God did not build you or many other people with the necessary brain material to make changes. Or you may think you just lack the neural tools to make the right lifestyle work. As with the Canadian study and many other ones, the data actually reveals that you might be right—for now.

The lack of time, discipline, motivation, will-power, good genetics, fast metabolism, functioning joints, caring, health, energy, money, support, and/or optimal digestion that has been, or you believe has been, stopping you may *not* be something you can just get over, as most of the self-help and diet gurus say you should.

What neuroscience now tells us is that the brain may be molded in such a way as to stop progress in its tracks. Therefore, it may not work long-term for you to just white-knuckle your way through life, or grin and bear it as you force yourself to run another five minutes on the tread-mill, or determine to kill the carbs or suck down that green drink. You may have to change your brain.

How to Grow a New Healthy Brain

While it may be true that you lack the brain you need, you can always build a new one! We all can think, plan, and act better than we are right now.

The key to good neuroplasticity is healthy use. These nerve connections, and their formations and reformations are due to lifestyle behaviors or the environment to which your brain is exposed. The more rich and positive that environment is, the better and better the brain can become.

Ways to Create Positive Neuroplasticity:

- Exercise
- Sleep
- A chiropractic adjustment

- Healthy fats: fish, flax, chia, hemp, coconut, olive, and avocado oils
- Green vegetables
- Berries
- Naturally raised animal proteins
- Meditation
- Healthy social relationships
- Coordinated, complex, cognitive activities: chess, playing the violin, crossword puzzles, working the computer keyboard, tai chi, yoga, learning sign language or Morse Code, sports

All of these can positively influence brain structures such as the all-important prefrontal cortex sitting there in the organism's Oval Office.

Ways to Create Negative Neuroplasticity:

- Stress
- Being too sedentary
- Processed or excessive carbohydrates
- Sugar
- Bad fats
- Commercial meat and dairy
- Subluxated spine and stiff, deconditioned muscles

CHANGE IS POSSIBLE

Like the old milk commercial used to say, "There's a new you coming every day." But it's not a newer, better you if your brain isn't "rewired."

Rewiring Time

Habits are formed in the brain because, as research indicates, the nervous system has an innate ability to heal, learn, and adapt (habituate) to common conditions. It also has the capacity to change or heal itself by recognizing patterns that are damaging and are causing chronic disease states. When it does, it then make important changes to help the organism (you) survive.

Studies also suggest that you can "dishabituate," or change your habits by reversing the brain's response or sensitivity to certain stimulations, such as a type of food or the repulsive thought of lifting weights. I call this "re-wiring."

The longer that your brain's "wiring" has been in place, the harder it is to change it. So when that new diet program clashes with the programming that is already in place in your brain, guess what? New diet loses. The good news is that, given time, the new programming becomes more permanent than the old programming and it's the bad habits that don't stick and have trouble coming back.

The more you repeat a behavior or an experience, the more fixed the wiring in your brain becomes. So when we talk about really changing a habit, we are talking about changing the wiring of the brain. But the brain doesn't rewire instantly. It requires time and repetition. The process goes like this: create the new wiring and then re-experience, re-experience, re-experience until the new wiring becomes more fixed in place than the old wiring.

In other words, when you go to CrossFit a few times, you are laying down new wiring. But you are also likely, at first, to back off or quit for any number of reasons people normally do: it's inconvenient, painful, makes you sore, boring, you hate all people that like working out, sweating sucks, you do not like messing up your hair and make-up, or the very thought or suggestion of exercise makes you want to vomit. You go back to the path of least resistance which is the old, existing wiring.

Nonetheless, as you re-experience, re-experience, re-experience the process, you start to enjoy the benefits, such as the endorphins, increased level of energy, more positive mental state, reduced need for medication, tighter buns and thighs, and so on. New structures are laid in place, and new wiring is secured.

As a result of this rewiring, believe it or not, you can become someone who cannot stand to miss a workout, is nauseated by the smell of fast food, now hates the sugar rush of soft drinks, loves salads, and seeks to avoid the hangover feeling because you're now too addicted to feeling good. The new habit becomes fixed.

Another example is one of our eating tricks, called the "Food Dress-Up Rule." I'll talk more about this in Chapter 6. The idea here is that you keep adding enough ingredients to vegetables, salads, or smoothies until you finally like them. And now that you actually like them, your thought-wiring about them changes over time as you learn to buy, use, prepare, and eat these foods,. Eventually, you might actually become someone who likes these foods so much that you enjoy eating them with less dressing-up.

The Food Dress-Up Rule enables your thoughts to be reconstructed, permitting a new habit to take hold from rewiring your brain. Trying to force new programs without the rewiring results in yo-yo dieting, gyms you never go to but ding your credit card for every month, a closet full of active-wear you never wear, and exercise equipment in your bedroom that has become an expensive towel rack or place to stack books.

Ultimately, it all works together: better habits give you a newer, better brain and over time, the brain provides newer, better habits.

Rewire the Brain and Reconstruct the Thoughts

Like the MRIs and the EEGs show us, our brain machine is wired to generate behavior and response to the environmental stimuli we encounter. For instance, as I shared:

The prefrontal cortex plays a major role in the strategic decision for the organism to pass or to choose better—like when you come face to face with a jelly donut!

When we see a picture, we fire off the occipital, visual portion of our brain.

If it's a sad picture we see or one that challenges our beliefs, the amygdala kicks in, responding to emotions, threats, and the subsequent decisions we will make in response.

Yet, there is also what philosopher Gilbert Ryle referred to as "the ghost in the machine." When your brain machine pushes out a response, you also contain the ability to think through it. As human beings, we do not have to do something dumb or behave in a destructive manner just because it is programmed in us.

Just as the brain pushes information out to the mind, so thoughts harness the brain's circuitry to enable us to explore ideas, choose a path, and change. It is a two-way street, and therefore as we are growing and remolding our new brain, we need to also lay hold of our thoughts.

Where the brain and its decision-making ability can be improved (plasticity) and its circuitry rewired, our thoughts also can be reconstructed to better suit our future. The fascinating duality here is that neuroplasticity improves our thoughts and mindful thought-improvement aids neuroplasticity. Wow!

Back to the Future

When that future fails to transpire on a continuing basis, it can be very detrimental to mental health. Famed Swiss psychologist Carl Jung said, "What you resist, persists, and what you give energy to manifests." Jung discovered that when people resisted certain aspects or parts of themselves, those aspects and parts not only persisted, they also enlarged. This process then draws even more energy into the resistance, which, again, causes resistance to enlarge. Ultimately, Jung was concerned about how this cycle could fracture the psyche, fragment the person, and draw them away from the kind of wholeness that is the substance of a satisfying existence.

For example, as you fight a craving and lament your lifestyle, the problem persists and grows stronger. It gets harder and harder to diet, work-out, meditate, or read. This makes it harder for you to grow into the kind of person you desire to be. Over time, you can grow to dislike parts of yourself, become disappointed, and—after having broken so many self-promises—stop trusting in yourself.

Viktor Frankl, the Holocaust survivor and author of the perennial best-selling book *Man's Search for Meaning*, found that we have to be living the story of our dreams or we'll instead create the pain and fragmentation that Jung warned us of. Your plan then, moving forward, is to stop resisting your biological cravings and shift your energy to a brain that is working for you, not against you, and establish an improved way of thinking. The results will be better than just another desperate attempt at resisting pasta! They will be about manifesting a new you.

Dr. Frankl found that, as humans, we require the freedom "to will." He described freedom as the ability to shape your life. He found that we need not only to be free, but also free to be and do something, or what he called the "will to meaning." We need to be able to achieve our desired goals and purposes and find meaning in our lives. His work, called Logotherapy, acknowledges that life is not some illusion that arises from a bunch of neurons and chemicals colliding together; rather, it's something with value that's worth experiencing to its fullest extent. If freedom of will, will to meaning, or life itself is limited, then we become stressed, depressed, or even hopeless and lost.

The good news is, as your brain and your thoughts proceed in a better direction, your story can change.

"There is no tomorrow!" —Apollo Creed ("The Count of Monte Fisto"), Rocky III

To win the inside battle of wellness, we have to learn how to do what is called *metacognition*, or learn how to "think about thinking." For example, it is often said, "Getting there is half the battle." However, when it comes to exercising, as

I have found from talking to thousands of people, it's more like three-quarters of the battle. The problem generally is getting outside of or above the thoughts going through your head that convince you to be a no-show to the day's fitness plan.

Most people tell me they are not strangers to doing some hard exercise, normally do not really mind it, and definitely want the results. The challenge is of course, motivating oneself.

I spoke to a client recently with a very common story. He was an athlete in high school, but since graduating he has an overwhelming amount of trouble getting himself to do any exercise. He genuinely dislikes how he looks and feels. His body image has snafued his confidence and really caused him to struggle to make friends and get dates. He wants to get his body back and can sometimes motivate for a week or two, but inevitably he then misses workouts for the next six months.

My question to him was, "What does the conversation sound like in your head when the inside battle to exercise starts?"

He gave me the fairly standard, vague answer: "I'm not sure. I want to do it, but there can be many things that enable me to talk myself out of it. Excuses pop up, like, 'It will be boring or painful. I feel tired. I do not feel up to it. I don't have the time.' Or I'll think about the future and decide I do not want to deal with the soreness the next few days."

I asked him, "What happens once you get to the gym?"

"Once I'm there and get going," he responded, "I do not mind the workout and I feel really good about myself after it is done."

These preworkout thought-skirmishes are so common that I timed them and named them. I call the time from when you know you should work-out to the time you are actually exercising *2 minutes and 45 seconds of hell* (or, 2/45). There is no way around it. The mental distance from Point A—where you are lying in your bed, or sitting on your couch, at your desk, or in the car—to Point B, when you are working out, can be hell.

But if you can learn to *think about your thinking* and realize the pain of showing up is short and the pain of skipping is really, really long, then you can push through it, more times than not. As I'll show you, the hell of it really never disappears completely, but with rewired thinking it is easier to win and win more often.

Anyone who knows me would call me a workout or fitness freak. I work-out five or six days each week. But what they don't know is what goes on in my head during my own 2/45.

Before one of my recent workouts, I was tired, sore, and a great college-football bowl game was on TV. My plan was to go for a run. I was lying on the floor inside my home to stretch. As soon as my back touched the carpet, the contrast between nap and exercise kicked into high gear and my inner voice started screaming: "*Nap wins, nap wins!*" Falling asleep right there on the floor suddenly felt like it would have qualified as the most incredible experience of my life. Better than marriage, kids, and when I won my first wrestling match. I thought, *I can sleep, wake up to watch the game, and spend the afternoon eating while sitting in my favorite chair, and always run tomorrow.*

Having been disappointed from losing this inside thought-battle many times, I knew better. My metacognition kicked in. Using a line that boxing champ Apollo Creed said to Rocky in *Rocky III* when Rocky wanted to put off his training to the next day, I said to myself using my best Carl Weathers impression: *There is no tomorrow!* Then, reluctantly, I took those first few steps down the road. About two minutes into the run, I was awake, warmed up, into it, and really glad I didn't take a nap.

Afterward, as is always the case, I felt good from the combination of endorphins and gratitude that I had accomplished something positive. A much better state of mind than the remorse that would've kicked in had I lost the inside battle to eleven minutes of sleep and the Las Vegas Bowl—which was being played two weeks before the real bowl games that did not occur until New Year's Day.

That 2 minutes and 45 seconds between Point A and Point B can be a losing battle for many, if not most people. A quick secret is just to think about your thinking and work on pushing through that 165 seconds. Showing up is 75+ percent of the battle! If you can just get to that point of motion, you'll do something—and something is better and more rewarding than nothing. "There is no tomorrow!"

Rewiring and thinking about your thinking will not eliminate all conflicting thoughts and excuses. We all make poor decisions, but we can choose to keep moving forward.

MINDFUL OF SUCCESS OR FAILURE

In a study called "Mindless Eating," published in the journal *Environment and Behavior*, authors Brian Wansinski and Jeffery Sobal sought to determine how many food decisions college students made in a day.[3] Of the 154 students they studied, the average response was 14.4 a day. However, when the factors of who, what, when, and where were added in, the number went up parabolically.

Questions such as, "Who did you eat with? What did you eat and how much? When did you decide to eat? When did you decide to stop eating? Where did you eat?" and so on, raised the average food decisions to 226.7 times per day. While this number may be inflated for effect, the point is clear: when it comes to your nutrition, there is a whole lot more to be mindful of than you're likely considering.

Like metacognition, the concept of *mindfulness* is an increased sensitivity to what is happening around you. In mindfulness, information comes into our conscious attention. As we awaken and begin to reflect on our choices, what is happening to our bodies, and how we are impacting the environment around us, change becomes possible.

As neuroplasticity improved the health of the entire brain, so mindfulness improves our entire person. Overall body function, immunity, healing, stress management, and sense of wellness are all beneficiaries of paying attention.

If you ever lived in a newly built house or apartment, you may have had to live with the side-effects of poor construction. The prestigious community of Lake Butler Sound, Florida, is around the corner from my home. This neighborhood of the rich and famous is the location of at least two homes where the owners over-reached and the houses have sat vacant for years. A leaky roof or windows, cracks in the foundation, plumbing problems, faulty wiring, and many other problems caused these money pits to fail to become someone's home. Despite the ornate designs, the bombastic landscape, the materials imported from all over the world, and the enormity of the investment, faulty construction killed the splendid plans.

Poor thought construction works the same way. Whether you are trying to succeed with the Paleo Diet, Weight Watchers, Atkins, Jenny Craig, biking, running, the gym, or a hundred other types of diet and exercise regimens, mindfulness and cognition must improve to see improvements, regardless of the program.

A Person of Conscience

My hope is that I will help you become a person who lives life "awake." I want to see you become someone who is thinking—and thinking about your thinking—and to help you eliminate not only mindless eating, but also anything else you may mindlessly do to your body. I want to help you become *a person of conscience.* Starting and sticking to anything important requires a conscious, intentional plan in which you are really thinking about the ROI (Return On Investment).

For any investment we make (unless it's a minimally-thought-out bad investment!), we have to consider the risks, the downsides, and true pay-offs of our decision. The same holds true for decisions we make about our eating. Personally, I am able to pass on many delicious-looking desserts, great-smelling breads, and caffeine cravings because when I consider the end game, it does not look good. After the brief joy of consumption, I know I'll be left with some level of a tummy ache, agitation, trouble sleeping (and more trouble getting up), and potentially a hefty dose of guilt.

That's why I always say that a McDonald's Happy Meal ultimately never made anyone very happy. It might be quick, cheap, tasty, and entertaining now, but the long-term ROI is that the happy turns to sad. Sooner or later it's an Unhappy Meal.

I have found that with people who really struggle from the continual intake of the wrong kinds of foods that there's often not enough thought going into their decisions. One of the Tricks I'll cover in Chapter 6 is to show you how to take Vacation Meals. These are the ones when you eat the pasta, cheese cake, or other favorite food you cannot live without only at a specified time each week. Even the people with the greatest choice challenges are able to consciously wait to eat these richer foods until Friday at lunch or Saturday dinner and avoid unconsciously risking their lives by eating them all the time or even randomly throughout a day or week.

You want to be a person of conscience, one who is mindful, or aware of the choices you make, for the sake of your health and appearance. Did you know the candies you see near store cash registers are called "impulse buys?" Merchants count on the fact that the overwhelmed human species will robotically purchase and consume toxic sugar gut-bombs while waiting at the checkout counter. I'm going to provide several methods, like Vacation Meals. that will help you not to be an impulse buyer. Let someone else buy the gum, the gobstopper, or the Hershey's bar from the trap next to the register, but not you.

"Diet is Die with a 't!" —Garfield (the cat, not the president)

When I speak at seminars and conferences, one topic that is always sure to get a visceral response from the audience is "diet books." I'll ask the crowd:

"How many of you have at least two diet books in your house right now?" (Every hand goes up.)

Then I ask, "How many of you have an entire diet-book library at your house?" (Many hands go up, and I hear a few laughs.)

Finally, I ask: "How many of you are still following any of the diet books or plans you have in your house?" (No hands go up, and I hear some light groaning.)

We don't need the results of research studies to know the world has gotten way out of shape—although it hasn't been caused by a lack of trying. People buy millions of books, CDs, and downloads every year related to health, fitness, and diet. It is likely that you or someone you know has one of *my* diet and fitness books in your library that was also unfinished, or even unopened. Unfortunately, as my informal crowd surveys show, though plenty of people buy better-lifestyle plans, most quit or never even start them. In fact, a UCLA study showed that while some diets can help you lose 5 percent to 10 percent of your weight, the pounds come right back—regardless of the type of book or diet plan, or which celebrity was on the cover.

There might be a hundred reasons so few people ever really reach their weight, health, and fitness goals. We find it so difficult, in fact, that we spend billions on surgeries, drugs, and other very expensive and extreme measures, all in an attempt to look better. Even when these costly, severe methods "work," the failure to combine them with substantive-enough life changes halts progress. Often, in fact, people's conditions revert to their previous states, or become worse.

Whether you need to lose weight for clinical/health purposes, just want to get into a smaller dress or pant size, are very overweight, want to retain your youth and energy, want to be in actual good shape, or want a six pack and a hot butt, the journey to a success result has certainly become paramount to climbing Mount Everest or swimming with a Great White shark. Few people can ever pull it off, it's very painful, and many have died trying!

At the risk of pointing out the obvious, I'll state it again: our wiring and thinking, when it comes to lifestyle change, is utterly broken. After decades of witnessing the failed wellness revolution, I saw clearly that I needed to tackle what is going on between our ears and give you a strategy to counter its role in stopping us from succeeding.

Your Thought Construction

I once saw an episode of a TV show in which two overweight actors played a couple who were desperately trying to lose weight. The writers made sure that the viewer realized the two characters hated every second of the process. In one scene, as they were walking out of the gym together, the male turned and screamed to all of the people behind him pumping iron and jogging on treadmills, *"This is the worst place in the world!"*

Although I wouldn't have called it the actual "worst place in the world," I certainly used to dread going to the gym. I would go because I liked the results, but I did not want to go. I used to think I was a Fruity Pebbles, pizza, and ice cream person who really hated exercise. Early on, my only health moments were my "shouldn'ts" and "shoulds"—I knew I *shouldn't* eat those foods and I *should* work out. Several days each month, and when I was really pushing myself, I'd grit my teeth, and with every ounce of determination I had, I'd eat something healthy or do some pushups.

Even while I was getting my nutrition degree, it was my sincere belief that pizza was not a want, but a need—that somehow pizza was a biological requirement for human survival and therefore my weekly consumption of it was a matter of life or death. That is how I was wired.

Now, however, I figuratively and literally love the gym. One of my favorite parts of being away at a nice hotel for a vacation or a seminar is the additional time I have to be in the fitness facility. I love to check out a new variety of equipment. When my assistant makes my reservation, she knows the most important question is to find out if the facility has a decent gym. No gym or bad gym = no reservation! My wiring changed, and I've seen it change in thousands of other people.

RECONSTRUCT THINKING TO DECONSTRUCT OLD HABITS

By breaking from habits related to our cognitive wiring and biases, we are able to form new opinions about ourselves and radically improve our chances for the life we want. Duke University researchers conducted a study, published in the *Journal of Neuroscience*, about habit formation, in which mice were trained to press a lever in order to receive a sugary pellet.[4] When the supply of these treats was later stopped, some mice continued to press the lever. Those mice had formed a habit. Now they were so hard-structured to getting sugar that they were going to press that darn lever until that dumb machine spit them out another Milky Way.

The fact that construction locks in our habits can be both good and bad news. The bad news for me was that I was not mentally built to be a health-conscious person. The repetition of my upbringing constructed in all-you-can-eat buffets, Fruity Pebbles, TV, ice cream *every* night, and short-term commitments to better habits. The good news for you and me is that we all can be reconstructed.

For us, the "lever" is often the context in which we are faced with a decision, or our environment. For example, I never think of popcorn except when I am…guess where? If you said, "Movies," you got it right. The movie lever can trigger popcorn, candy, and a soft drink. It also brings up another well-studied context, which relates to serving size. Research shows that if you get a small bag of popcorn, you will eat a small bag of popcorn.[5] But at the movies, you order the bucket—so you eat a bucket.

Buffets, favorite restaurants, drinking buddies, tailgating, movies, foodie friends, and other pleasures you surround yourself with that inspire habits contrary to the lifestyle you're attempting to create are potential levers. They're therefore relevant to this concept of context. Be mindful of the levers in your life as you look to reconstruct your thinking and deconstruct old habits.

Thoughts Behind Our Addictions

Food is a drug of choice for so many of us. Personally, I'm a stress eater. Research on stress and eating shows that overindulging acts just like a drug in responding to the brain, glands, and hormone stress cycle. So effectively, I'm a drug addict.

Substance addiction has been an insidious, ubiquitous condition throughout the history of the world. It destroys lives and families, and influences the success of entire cultures. There are a complexity of issues that cause at least 1 in 10 people to struggle with it. The numbers would be much higher if they included addiction to carbs.

It is a well-known scientific fact that the overconsumption of drugs and alcohol leads to more serious problems. The same is true of being overweight—even on a moderate scale. Being modestly overweight increases the risk of dying of all causes, and even moderate drinking creates an increased risk of cancers such as breast cancer, oral cancer, and colon cancer.[6] The point here is that these facts do not necessarily deter people from eating poorly or getting drunk. That is the power of addiction.

Positive-Incentive Value of Addiction

Whether the substance is a drug, a drink, or a food, a major part of the challenge to reversing addiction is that the substance is addictive in a threefold way: physically, emotionally, and socially. Helpful to our understanding the emotional connection to addiction is knowing that just the thought of the involved substance can trigger a deep desire to consume it.

You'll learn in the Tricks and Secrets section in the last chapter that because I rarely eat anything bad, it no longer causes me any harm. Comfort foods for me are grain-free, sugar-free desserts and almond crusted pizza. So there are no negative side-effects. When my comfort food used to be ice cream, stress eating was a real problem.

This is a thought-construction side of addiction called "positive-incentive value." This rationale states that people become addicted in the anticipation of the pleasure they will experience as a result of the substance of choice and not because of the Hedonic value of the substance, which is the actual pleasure it can bring.

The anticipated, positive-incentive value is so strong that even when the Hedonic value does not exist and someone is no longer enjoying a drug, they may still desire it. This can explain how a food, drink, or a drug can be destroying someone's life, causing incredible physical and emotional pain, yet the individual remains addicted. Like all constructed thoughts, positive-incentive value increases with time and repetition until the cravings override any of the negative effects.

Food does not cause what is considered true physical dependence. Instead, dependence results from the chronic reward process, as we saw with the mouse, the lever, and the sugar pellets. Meaning that: I eat the carbs, create pleasure thoughts, and repeat until eventually my mind ends up pretty focused on the *desire* for carbs.

Reversing Positive-Incentive Value

Craving negative rewards such as sugar or the mindless state of a drunken stupor are what noted behavioral psychologist B.F. Skinner called "conditioning." Conditioning, good or bad, occurs through repetition. Poor conditioning sets you up lifestyle relapse. Thankfully, through more constructive repetitions, this process also work in reverse and eventually sets you up for successful maintenance of the life you want to live.

We, not unlike the mouse, also develop our habits based on rewards from our environment. I desire love, and I notice that when I smile and treat people nicely I receive love—so I smile and treat people nicely. My work pays me money, which I need, and I learn from my environment that when I work harder, I get paid more. Thus, I develop a stronger work ethic.

Some people, when thinking of exercise, are conditioned to feel terror. Others are attracted by or even addicted to the positive reward. The positive-incentive value of exercising is that it creates a better appearance and the constructive feeling of accomplishment at the end of the workout. Environment teaches you that the more you exercise, the better you will look and feel until, ultimately, a habit is born.

I have strong contextual cues when it comes to getting up to work-out in the morning. The best time to exercise is in the morning before breakfast, but when the alarm goes off I always have an excuse at the ready to hit snooze. While it is *always* difficult, I know the reward I'll receive from the workout. It will put me in a positive place physically and mentally the rest of the day and beyond. That is way better than the reward the nine extra minutes of sleep supplies.

Positive-incentive value works the same for me when it comes to the topic of fresh bread or rich desserts. Those foods get every one of my five senses going It *looks, sounds,* and *smells* so good, I can almost *feel* the texture in my mouth and *hear* myself saying, "Wow—that's awesome." I have reversed this over time by knowing that this environment kicks back something else. I feel lousy physically and mentally after consuming these super-dense carbs, and so the real reward is getting past the craving and feeling good, and good about myself later.

I also know I can make it home and eat one of the many grain-free, sugar free desserts that have 80 percent of the pleasure and 0 percent of the pain and regret.

THE TRUTH ABOUT HUNGER (HINT: IT'S MORE BRAIN THAN BELLY.)

The desire to eat, which we call "hunger," is normally attributed to a need for energy the body requires in order for it to return back to ideal levels—back to the energy "set-point."

The assumption is that after you eat and restore optimum energy levels, they start to decline until they have dropped below a certain point, at which time hunger kicks in and calls out for more food. You then eat until you're back again to optimum; the cut-off is triggered by feeling satisfied or full.

However, the set-point theory has been disproved through the mass of evidence that has come out since its inception in the 1990s. It has failed to hold up because the drop in glucose would have to be enormous in order to induce the desire to eat—well beyond what ever normally occurs in the body. Additionally, the average person has substantial fat stores that could be utilized for energy; so it's not like you were going to die if you didn't eat lunch. That's because negative-feedback systems are designed to create homeostasis and stabilize the body's internal environment.

What actually initiates the feeling of hunger are things like taste, learning, and outside influences. When you think of food, especially super-rich and delicious food, it triggers the desire for it in the absence of any kind of need. If you know that dinner happens at 6 p.m. or 7 p.m., then that is far more likely to be the reason for eating at that time than any kind of actual nutrient deficiency.[7]

It may really blow your mind to know that the concept of hunger = pain from an empty stomach/satisfaction = a full stomach has been totally disproved. When people have their stomachs surgically removed, hooking their esophagus up directly with the small intestine, they continue to report feeling hungry or satisfied.

As it is with drug and alcohol consumption, positive-incentive value is the most likely reason for eating and the sensation of hunger. We are hungry and drawn to indulge due to the anticipated pleasure and not the actual need, deficit, or true reward. Hunger is essentially like sex. We don't jump in because of a sex-deficit; we do it because we crave it. And like with food, some people really regret it later!

The body actually learns to be hungry. The studies show that when the usual meal time approaches, the body takes measures to prepare for the influx of food. My dogs do the same thing; they start circling their bowls at the precise time we feed them every day.

The research reveals what may seem like a shocking conclusion: the unpleasant feeling of hunger you experience before eating is not due to your body's desire to be fed; it's due to the disturbances within your body as it prepares for digestion.

4 Tricks to Take Away From "The Truth About Hunger":

If you follow our Stay Full Rule in Chapter 6, then your pre-meal, hunger-preparation effect will not be as strong.

Avoid the Appetizer Effect[8] and the Cafeteria Diet.[9] Variety kills volume control. It starts and restarts the positive-incentive value and bypasses your body's satiety resources. Variety makes you eat more!

Take advantage of Sensory-Specific Satiety.[10] When you fill up on one dish rather than having an appetizer first, or when you avoid the context of a cafeteria or buffet with their multitude of options, your desire to eat more drops considerably. More on this in Chapter 6 as part of the 10-Point Reduction Rule.

The preparation for digestion-induced hunger that kicks in because the body knows it is getting close to feeding time eventually goes away if the meal is not served. People who do fasting or intermittent fasting will tell you that the hunger pains drop off fairly quickly when ignored.

chapter 3

A BEAUTIFUL MIND

THE COUNTER

A FTER READING THE BOOK SO far, you might be saying, "Great, Dr. Ben—this might work for some people, but you don't understand *my situation*."

As someone who wrestled competitively for nineteen years, I understand completely what it's like to be caught in a dangerous, painful condition from which it appears impossible to wriggle free. If you're tired enough, hurting enough, behind by enough points, and have been working hard to no avail for a long enough time, the thought of success can all but completely diminish—and cease even being a dream. In an exhausted, unmotivated, painful state, all that may seem reasonable at that point are antidepressants, alcohol, or a whole lot of sugar. But there is a better, less harmful way.

In wrestling, there are certain positions or "holds" that you never want to find yourself in. Getting caught in a "cradle," "guillotine," "double chicken wing," or being stuck on your back all are potentially dangerous, match-ending states of affair. In fact, if your opponent is really good, it can seem like there's no way out of his hold, and an "all is lost" feeling of discouragement and despair can come over you pretty quickly. However, the truth is, there's always a way out. That's why many wrestlers have broken these holds, fought successfully to get off their backs, and come back to win their matches.

These winners knew something very important: *They knew how to counter.*

As boxed in as you may feel now; as much as you may feel like, "It's over," and that you're at the end of your rope, *don't quit.* Instead, *counter.* The *counter* is how you escape and come back from a compromising position. It applies not only to an athletic wrestling match but also to life's wrestling matches.

HOW TO COUNTER

Here are three ways to successfully counter when you feel like your lifestyle has you locked up and down for the count:

1. Change your position. You have to be capable of seeing outside of your box of frustration and become aware of your blind spots. Death is in the blind spots. They're so big you can fit an invisible eighteen-wheeler into one! In the world of success, as futurist author Alvin Toffler said, "The illiterate are not people who can't read or write; they're the ones can't *learn, unlearn,* and *relearn.*"

2. Get mad instead of sad! To successfully counter, you have to get mad instead of sad. You need some tacking fuel! Use the fuel of failure as energy instead of despair, and you'll muster up more strength than you believed you had. Your mind always quits before your body. You can keep going.

3. *Want it—bad!* When you first start wrestling, you stink at it and need to know a lot of counters. When I asked my coach how to get out of some of the more compromising positions, he said, "If you want to get out, it's got to be like you're a drowning man trying to come up for air." Make it like a purpose you would die for. You have to want it bad!

Winning the Battle and the War

The information here is not designed to be or replace your psychotherapist. It is meant to bubble to the surface of your perceptions and lift your decision making up to a level of mindful awareness. If you can begin to know your mind better and where thoughts and beliefs are coming from, then you can become more fully conscious of your decision making. Whether you decide to choose the ideal decision for your body or not, I think you'd agree that you should at least be *awake* for these decisions as you make them.

Cognitive psychology is a study of how information is processed when it is received by your brain and how you use it to solve problems and make decisions. Our responses are not as simplistic as some amoebic or snail-like behavioral reflex to external stimuli. Experiences and information trigger emotions in a moment, based on whatever meaning you assign to them.

Our human tendency is to assume that we all react similarly to stress and circumstances and feel the same way about what comes our way. But, in reality, the emotions you assign to the information coming in can be radically different from what I or others assign to them. If they can be different, then they can also be better. Doesn't it make sense to improve how you react to life in order to get the best results possible for yourself and your family?

Our assessments of emotion-stimulating events, as well as our responses to them, can happen at a conscious or unconscious level. By thinking about how we think, we can learn and predict these responses and start to really know our inner selves. Without this self-knowledge, your life can really be like a boat lost at sea with no oars or motor. The wind, the sea, the currents, and the fish are in charge. Any time circumstances are in charge of you, it makes for a tough trip.

British psychologist, Frederick Bartlett found that memory does not work simply through experience, as most people assume. Instead, the mind constructs and reconstructs the data coming in and creates its own biased interpretations. It isn't really what you specifically have seen, heard, and tasted that matters as much as what you made of it all.

So if you have decided that exercise is the worst and sleeping in and eating waffles for breakfast are the best, then that is simply a framework or perception you have constructed. Someone who hates exercise and loves waffles but works out anyway and eats eggs instead has constructed something else. Bartlett found that people stuck in unhealthy "schemas," or habits, have embellished or trumped up the memories of events to make them seem so desirable that they just can't resist living them out.

A memory or a thought is actually something people construct in such a way as to satisfy their own impressions or prejudices relative to the actual event. There is scripture that says, "As [a person] thinks in his heart, so is he" (Prov. 23:7, NKJV). It says *as* a person thinks rather than *what* he thinks. As a consultant, physician, and coach I have come to understand that how you process information or think, unlearn, and relearn is critical to growth.

Here are some great examples of biased perceptions from history. As you'll see, each statement was way off!

FAMOUS FIRST WORDS

"Man will never reach the moon, regardless of all future scientific advances." —*Dr. Lee DeForest, a father of radio | Feb. 25, 1957*

"Airplanes are interesting toys but of no military value." —*Marshall Ferdinand, FOCH, French military strategist and World War 1 commander | 1911*

"Everything that can be invented has been invented." —*Charles H. Duell, U.S. Commissioner of Patents | 1899*

"We don't like their sound. Groups of guitars are on the way out." —*Decca Records executive, upon rejecting a contract with the Beatles*

"He is not very talented." —*Albert Einstein's elementary school teacher*

"Stocks have reached what looks like a permanently high plateau." —*Irving Fisher, professor of economics, Yale University | October 1929*

"I have no political ambitions for myself or my children." —*Joseph P. Kennedy | 1936*

"I think there is a world market for maybe five computers." —*Thomas Watson, president of IBM | 1943*

"Television won't be able to hold on to any market it captures after the first six months. People will soon get tired of staring at a plywood box every night." —*Darryl F. Zanuck, studio executive, Twentieth-Century Fox Film Corp. | 1946*

"There is no reason for any individual to have a computer in their home." —*Kenneth Olsen, president and founder of Digital Equipment Corp. | 1977*

"Vitamins give you expensive urine." —*Medicine's early opinion on supplementation*

"There is no harm to GMOs, amalgam fillings, medications, food additives, artificial sweeteners, or smoking and drinking in moderation." —*Said by most anyone who profits from these industries*

THE WAY WE SEE THE WORLD

In 1941 and 1942, Jews in most parts of Europe were forced to wear the Star of David. This was required by the Nazis as a way to label them and hold them to a set of restrictions. With no laws in place to protect Jews, violating a restriction could mean severe punishment or death. The rules included a strict 6 p.m. curfew.

When Daniel Kahneman, an award-winning economist and psychologist, was only seven or eight years old, he had gone to play with a Christian friend and failed to realize that he had stayed out past curfew. In an effort to get home safely, he turned his sweater inside out, attempting to hide his star and headed home hoping to avoid trouble. As he was traveling down an empty street, he saw a German soldier in a black uniform approaching him. Specially recruited SS soldiers wore the black uniforms and were the men that children were taught to fear most. Kahneman tried to walk quickly by him, but the soldier called him over.

Rather than arresting him, however the soldier hugged him, showed him a picture of his own son who was of the same age, and gave him some money. Kahneman saw that there are compassionate people in some of the most horrifying places and spaces, and this verified to him that different people are conditioned to have very diverse views of the world.

Later in his life, Kahneman coined the term "heuristics," which refers to the rules of thumb we accept, such as a broadly accepted guide or principle based on one's experience or practice. He came to these conclusions when he discovered what he called the "illusion of validity." This is a tendency for people to view their own beliefs as reality, even though in many, if not most, cases there is plenty of evidence to the contrary. If someone's "heuristics" are locked in tightly enough, then even when faced with the facts they will filter out reality and stick to their opinions.

We tend to just believe in what we know from our own point of view and set of experiences. Unfortunately, those beliefs can be strongly limited or even dead wrong. These heuristics can trap you in the same place body, mind, and spirit if you do not learn to understand yours and make an effort to break free.

Previously, we worked through the important principles of thinking and awareness such as *mindfulness, metacognition, thinking about our thinking, unlearning,* and *relearning.* These principles will help us become aware of heuristic biases and learn how we learn.

BREAKING FREE FROM OUR LIMITED VIEW OF REALITY

Visible light is not the only source of illumination in the universe. Rather, it is a sliver of electromagnetic radiation made up of 400-700 nanometers (billionths of a meter). This is measured on the spectrum of gamma waves that are trillions of nanometers shorter than radio waves, which are trillions of nanometers longer. We are continually bathed in these electromagnetic rays, but without instrumentation we are totally oblivious to their existence because the human retina is designed to only see 400-700 nanometers.

Similarly, humans can hear only 20-20,000 hertz (Hz), which refers to cycles of compressed air per second. To hear beyond this range you have to be a dog; or be like bats, which send ultrasonic waves into the air and listen to them as they bounce off of prey so they can hone in and feed. Only through the use of new technology can scientists hear these bat sounds and track their movement.

Before the inventions of such technologies, mankind was clueless—literally blind to much of the light and deaf to much of what goes on in the world. The same blindness and deafness can prejudice us to the way we think the world works, how we view ourselves, and what we believe to be possible.

In a rational world, when given a choice, we would evaluate a probability and take note of all possible outcomes, combining all factors to make a judgment call. Unfortunately, we rarely have all the facts; it's not possible to know all the outcomes, and even if we were given all of that data, we do not possess enough mental flexibility, brain capacity, or time to analyze all of it. Instead, the decisions we make are based on our limitations. This refers to limitations of the brain, time constraints, and the partial information we know or have received.

Many of the decisions we make about the self, about self-discipline, and about what we think are appropriate choices for our body are majorly prejudiced by these underlying heuristic mental rules. Understanding some common heuristic biases and becoming aware of how they may be screwing up your life can change your future by helping you (remember this!): *Think, Unlearn,* and *Relearn.*

TYPES OF HEURISTIC BIASES
PRESENT BIAS

This one hits the bull's-eye when it comes to improving long-term commitment to anything, particularly wellness. *Present bias* is the inability to comprehend that what you want at this moment will be much different later.

What you want changes with time. I worked at a gym all through college. Our gym membership was a one-year contract for which fees were automatically transferred each month from a member's bank account to ours, starting the day you joined. On Sunday mornings, we would have dozens of people sign up for the year…and we would never see them again. They would not work-out or even use the option to take a free shower in the gym. Unless they had a coupon for a discount rate, they had just thrown away $600!

The gym membership is a great example of present bias. People would have a hard weekend of beer drinking, late-night eating, sleeping in, Mimosas, and Bloody Marys. They'd wake up Sunday morning looking like the Crypt Keeper or Jabba the Hutt and say: "That's it! I am never drinking again! I am going to start eating nothing but broccoli, and, darn it—I'm joining the gym!"

Present bias occurs when you order shoes or a blouse online that you never wear, sign up for a subscription to a magazine you never read, say yes to a date you later regret, or make a New Year's resolution you don't achieve. At the time you made those decisions, you were committed in that moment to follow through with what you'd chosen to do. However, you failed to consider how you might feel about it hours, days, weeks, or months later.

Present Bias Wellness Examples:

You step on the scale in the morning, hate what you see, and buy the exercise equipment right off the infomercial. You think, "This one looks like an exercise product I'd enjoy, and I won't have to leave the apartment to exercise." Now it's a week later, and the only way to fit the workout into your schedule is to get up eighteen minutes earlier. Instead, you hit the snooze button.

You are looking in the mirror while getting ready for school and you do not like what you see. You declare, "No more carbs, ever!" But you're at the movies a couple of days later, and the popcorn hits your senses and you feel differently about carbs now. You buy the bucket.

You and a friend agree at a party that you're going to start running together. "It is finally time," you say. Two days later the friend calls, and you opt out so you can watch your favorite old movie or Kardashian Family rerun. That, or you just don't have the motivation you had over cocktails at the party. Your initial enthusiasm is what we call, "cocktail talk."

Over the weekend, you committed to salads for lunch—all week. You look at the lunch menu on Tuesday, and the salad just doesn't seem like it's going to cut it. You go for the burger and fries.

At a recent party, several of my friends who like to drink came up with what at the time seemed like a brilliant idea to them—an app that helps you find people to drink with when you travel. The more beers they drank and the later it got, the bigger this app was going to be. There was even discussion on moving to St. John in the Caribbean to live in one of the mountain homes that overlooks the bay and have a private jet with the name of the app painted on the side.

The next day everyone figured out that a good app can cost $60,000-$100,000 to make, that there already were three popular apps that did the same thing, and that no one really was ready to stop his life to start the next "Facebook." The night before, the present bias of cocktail talk had kicked in. The dream was dead in less than twenty-four hours.

The moral of these biases is that we need to really think through and not dismiss these short circuits in our brain wiring and thought construction. Through awareness, you can start to make far more legitimate commitments.

The Dunning-Kruger Effect

Cognitive bias studies done by psychologists David Dunning and Justin Kruger discovered some of the principles underlying the armchair quarterback; armchair president of the United States; armchair CEO; and armchair coach, teacher, doctor, pastor, or any other leader.[1]

The phenomenon is called the Dunning-Kruger Effect, and it can really impact your lifestyle decision-making. It is the reality that less competent people rate their competence higher than it actually is, while more competent people humbly rate theirs lower than it actually is.

As it relates to transforming your body, it means...you think you know too much.

Most people have very strong opinions on what is good or bad for them. They know best what they are willing or not willing to eat—much like the child who just knows he will not like what Mom made for dinner. To which, moms around the world will say: "How do you know you won't like it? You have even tried it!" This is usually followed by, "You at least have to try a bite." If Mom is forceful enough, the child will take the bite (and then spit it out!).

Adults are the same way. They have locked in their opinion; they've closed down on a better possible future. A person on the wise side of the Dunning-Kruger phenomenon will not look at yesterday's habits and opinions about wellness and determine they already know how tomorrow is going to be.

The most competent approach is to stay open to better, newer maps and roadways that can take you down a better route to wellness.

OPTIMISM, PESSIMISM BIAS

People tend to have unrealistic optimism and overzealous pessimism. We tend to be too optimistic about our own abilities and unreasonably pessimistic about the possibilities that exist for the future—all at the same time. These two facts can totally derail your transformative attempts.

The Danger of Optimism

Dr. Viktor Frankl, the Holocaust survivor and founder of Logotherapy mentioned earlier, developed several theories about why certain prisoners perished while others survived the death camps of Nazi Germany. One of the consistent emotional patterns exhibited by those who did not make it was over-optimism. The prisoners who said, "I'll be home by Christmas," or, "This will be over by Valentine's Day," suffered the most. It's better to acknowledge when you are up against a formidable challenge and accept that you're in for what can be a bumpy rollercoaster of a ride.

The hardest patients to work with are those who focus on fast results rather than the process of getting well. Everyone enjoys a quick fix, but even for the best of us, cleaner living has its ups and downs. The best mind-set is to expect to fall or fail but trust that you can always get up and fail forward.

Books on positive mental attitude will tell you that you can create a new habit in twenty-one days. While there have been some early studies to support this, it is *overly optimistic.* You may have already figured that out for yourself. Creating new habits are just not that simple.

In research created at University College London, ninety-six subjects attempted to turn an everyday health-related behavior into a habit. It was discovered that the average amount of time it took to form a habit was 66 days. Although drinking a glass of water a day took only 20 days before the habit formed, the habit of adding fruit to the diet took twice as long. Adding exercise, as you might imagine, was the toughest. Habit formation ranged from 50 days to develop a 10-minute-a-day walking habit to 84 days for a 50-morning sit-ups routine. In analyzing the data, it is conceivable that for more intense habit change, it could take closer to one year.

As counterintuitive and anti-self-help as it may sound, it's better for you to stay a little pessimistic. Of colossal importance to your success is the recognition that authentic, long-term change can take time, and until those habits are locked in you will have lapses when you fail to comply. Yet, the study also revealed that falling off the plan for a day or two did not impact the ability to eventually create the habit. Pivotal to good results, then, is: (1) being more pessimistic in the short-term, (2) setting expectations that include set-backs and a longer time for new habit formation, and (3) not letting any of that deter you from working to create the new you.

Over-Confidence

With my weight-loss patients I have found it common that they feel confident they can get things done later. "Later" they will get back on track. The problem with getting back "on track" is that failing to get into shape may actually be on track for you. This means that when you're sleeping in and eating fries, that's when you are actually on track. To get healthy, then, you don't need to get on track; you actually need to get "off track"! "I'll pull it off later," is another part of the delusion of unrealistic optimism.

Procrastination: The Great Goal Killer

Procrastination is like reverse present bias: you don't feel like it presently, but you convince yourself you'll feel like it later. It is again an example of being overly optimistic.[2]

Procrastination is the gateway drug of quitting any commitment. You slip once; it's OK, though, because you're convinced you'll get back on track. You'll restart Monday. *This will be my last bad weekend*, you think. *I'll finish this carton of ice cream to get it out of the house and never buy any again.*

But as you slide more and more regularly, that day on which you made the commitment ends up lost in the rearview. Next thing you know, it's December again—and you decide you'll just party through the holidays and make the resolution again for the new year. And this year, you tell yourself convincingly, "I'm gonna do it!"

Pessimistic About the Future

The interesting antithesis to overzealous optimism is the accompanying overzealous pessimism about our future. The two walk hand in hand as failed, overly optimistic attempts to succeed. Eventually you begin to doubt that change and pleasant results are coming your way.

The theme for the 2012 London Summer Olympics was, "Amazing awaits." New habits do eventually form, and the future can be brighter than you could ask or imagine it to be—if you address both sides of this bias. Plan to fail and have a plan ready for when you do. Achieving any goal is wrought with ups and downs, but it is not hard to create a plan that can ultimately prevail. *Be a realist about the battle, but an optimist about winning the war.*

CONFIRMATION BIAS

Confirmation bias is our propensity to look for or interpret information in a way that confirms our preconceived notions.[3] We take on a biased search for information and favor only evidence that supports our opinion, regardless of the validity of the evidence. Example: "It's on the Internet so it must be true." Our interpretation of any information becomes biased according to whether it agrees or disagrees with our own pre-existing theories.

Confirmation bias makes absolutely certain you never expand your perspective or learn to benefit from new ones. This limits or eliminates your ability to take in the new data required to change from outdated opinions and improve your competency. Instead of expanding your horizons, you subconsciously look for media, people, books, or information that agrees with your perspective and notice anything that supports its reliability. By contrast, you notice every flaw in information that opposes your beliefs.

As an example, if you believe someone is greedy or self-serving, then you will resonate with others who feel the same way and perceive anything that person does as an example of their selfish, money-hungry self. Even if they donated a million dollars to the poor, you'd think it was an act or a PR scheme.

I know some fast-foodies who have a full-blown case of confirmation bias toward their bodies. They regularly eat at McDonald's and Taco Bell, they drink every night, and they are twenty-five to thirty pounds overweight. They hang out with people who live a very similar lifestyle and join them on their midnight McDonald's runs. As time has gone on, the extra weight has become weight they hate. Yet, when assessing their lifestyle, they confirm their position by pointing out people who eat even worse or drink even more. Thus, they confirm that their behavior is cool.

They have also substantiated that people who have the body they want and do take care of themselves are prudish, stiff, not-fun people. Everyone around them and everything they read is converted into information that confirms they are doing life the way life should be done. When they have their moments when their clothes don't fit, they briefly lament their decisions but quickly unconfirm the new thoughts and go out to buy some bigger clothes. (The reasoning? "I need a new wardrobe anyway!")

To address your confirmation bias, acknowledge that it is time to give the other side a chance, and expand your horizons. Because you can *mindfully think*, look for information that opposes your ideas and listen to the opinions of people who do not agree with you, and then analyze that data.

CULTURAL BIAS

In 1998, I was nutritionist and chiropractor for the U.S. World Greco-Roman Wrestling team. We competed at the World Championships in Gavle, Sweden. At the time, Sweden was the healthiest country in the world (America was then, and still is, at the bottom of the healthcare barrel). Thus, I was really excited not only to care for our team and help athletes win some medals, but also to learn more about what makes bodies in Sweden function so well.

Industrially, technologically, administratively, militarily, and financially the U.S. is the most advanced country on the planet today. We have all the good toys, which makes us the most powerful kid on the playground.

However, many of the same things that make us the greatest also make us the sickest. It is not just what we eat, what's missing from our food, what's been added to our water, or some special kind of vitamin or drug we are not taking that makes us so much sicker and unhappier than other counties. What has destroyed our health and our lives is our very culture itself. Our philosophy, how we act, and how we work and do business are significantly different from Europe's, particularly the planet's healthiest nation, Sweden.

The Garden of Sweden

Sweden actually shut down McDonald's. (Think about that!) While we were on our way from the airport to meet with the Olympians, our cab driver told us that McDonald's restaurants were shut down because their food was too high in fat. They forced Ronald McDonald to lower the fat content of all his foods and pull the fat out of the special sauce. Our cabbie then proceeded to give us a five-minute dissertation on the dangers of a diet too high in saturated fats. There are three points I found very significant here:

The driver was that passionately concerned about the health of his body.

The entire nation was concerned about health.

They cared so much, they were willing to do something about it and take massive action by actually taking on the Mickey D corp.

The reason we are so dramatically sicker in the U.S. compared with Scandinavian countries is based on cultural lifestyle biases. The "Garden of Sweden" culture is biased toward health. I am sure they have overweight people, but we did not see a single one during our entire trip. The food we saw was very whole, the "drug" stores had large signs on their windows about homeopathic and herbal remedies, people walked everywhere—to the extent that there is walking rush-hour traffic—the people sit down for long, slow meals together; the portions are much smaller; and the country fights companies that try to poison their food.

I had an intern from Sweden once who, after being in the states several years, had adapted to our culture. When his parents came to visit and saw the twelve-inch sub he ordered from Subway they thought something was wrong with him.

I speak and work with many minority cultures that, as a whole, often suffer from many of the same types of diseases. This has far less to do with genetics and more to do with the foods, drinks, and general norms related to the way their families do life together. The same cultural biases likely exist in your family that may be leading you down the road of some really bad habits and conditions.

In the book, *Tuesdays With Morrie* by Mitch Albom, Morrie tells us how to effectively break free from our destructive cultural biases: "If your culture isn't working out, create your own."

Another book, the Bible, talks about culture-limiting bias as well. God is the ultimate psychotherapist. In the case of Abram, God told him that he had to move out in order to be blessed and be a blessing to the world. God said to Abram, "Go forth from your country, and from your relatives, and from your father's house to the land which I will show you; and I will make you a great nation, and I will bless you, and make your name great; and so you shall be a blessing" (Gen. 12:1, NASB).

For Abram, God's reason for moving his physical location was not as much about a change in geography as a way to get him out of his cultural biases and open up a new way for him to do life so he could fulfill his destiny. Upon Abram's leaving, God changed fatherless Abram's name to *Abraham*, which means, "the father of many."

You may not need to change your name, but you may need to change your cultural biases in order to be transformed. "Leaving home" is a metaphor for getting unstuck from unhealthy connections that no longer are serving you or God's purposes very well.

HELPLESS BIAS

A Harvard study found that a great deal of cancer could be prevented by lifestyle. The study also concluded that if you got cancer, you had a good chance of overcoming it by correcting how you were living.

Harvard then conducted a survey to see how many people would believe the conclusions. In the survey, more than 50 percent of the people believed they were powerless to stop diseases like cancer from developing. They believed there was nothing they could change in their lifestyle to stop illness from happening and shortening their lives. Further, they thought that if they developed a disease, there was nothing they could do or change to help cure it or fight it off. Ultimately, half the people studied felt helpless against cancer.

The helpless bias commonly occurs when people (or animals) feel like they have no control over their situation or their destiny. Ultimately, they are inclined to give up and accept their fate. Also called, "learned helplessness," knowledge of this bias comes from experiments by positive psychologist Martin Seligman, who discovered that dogs that received unavoidable electric shocks failed to take action in subsequent situations in which escape or avoidance of the shocks was possible. On the other hand, he found that dogs that had not received the unavoidable shocks immediately took action in subsequent situations when shocks were applied.[4] (Yes, my two dogs and I agree—a terrible experiment!)

The helpless bias is why there is extreme danger in the overzealous explanation of the contribution of genes to health, body type, personality, and potential. When someone believes their future is out of their control, they often stop trying. Let's face it, it is easier to say there is nothing you can do than to have to take responsibility for your circumstances. But there is always something you can do. Despite evidence or bias to the contrary, you have something to say about your future.

Here's a short word-association test. If the first word makes you immediately think of the following word or sentence, then you are biased toward a desire to consume junk food.

Word Association Bias Test

- Car: drive-through
- Up: side-down cake
- Down: the hatch
- Light: on the mayo
- Morning: breakfast burrito
- Night: time snack
- Happy: Hour
- Dark: chocolate
- White: Castle
- Plop, plop, fizz, fizz: Alka-Seltzer

If you responded to any of the first words of the test with the second words, or if one or more of these biases describes you, then you could use some thought reconstructing. Obviously, we all can. And if you don't think this applies to you, you're biased!

THE NORMALCY BIAS

"Wake up to this bias if you want to live!" —CALIF. GOV. ARNOLD SCHWARZENEGGER

On her first patient appointment in my office, Clara, an emphysema sufferer, stood in the parking lot with her oxygen tank and tubes in her nose and, in the available face hole that was left, smoked a cigarette. We can see the same thing at any restaurant, movie theater, theme park, grocery store, convenience store, or county fair—people who even have weight extremes or health problems continuing to pour the abuse on their bodies. Chronic disease, obesity, and extremes of suffering are not enough to stop them from consuming supersize sodas, Slurpees, fries, and candy along with popcorn buckets, fried Oreos, caramel lattes, and anything else for sale that spends a moment on the lips and a lifetime on the hips (and arteries). After my mother's stroke, confirmed 100 percent by tests to have been caused by smoking, she could not wait to get out of the hospital to start smoking again.

Somehow the many sufferers of normalcy bias like Clara and my mom assume they can continue down a destructive path and, despite all evidence to the contrary, it will all be OK.

This seems completely ludicrous. But there is a known psychological phenomenon that describes this behavior. One theory of how people ignore statistics like these and continue to act in ways that put their lives at risk is the *normalcy bias*.[5]

It is a powerfully influential problem. In Florida, where I have lived the last twenty-five years, we have hurricane season. Unlike with the holiday season, most Florida residents enter hurricane season with fear and trepidation. The joke, though, is that hurricane and holiday seasons do have a few things in common: during both seasons the stores are packed, you stock up on food, you leave home to visit relatives, and eventually there's going to be a tree in your house.

Some years, it becomes clear that a coastal city is going to take a direct, dangerous, and devastating hit. With today's technology, meteorologists can provide information to local governments with ample forewarning to make sure people have time to secure their homes or, in the case of the bigger storms, *evacuate*. Despite these warnings, and even if law enforcement demands an evacuation, a fascinating and disturbing phenomenon occurs: *many people stay and do nothing*. Often they do so with catastrophic consequences. This decision too is often due to the normalcy bias.

Psychologists and sociologists have found normalcy bias to be an unfortunate part of human nature. It is generally seen as a state of denial many people exhibit when their lives are in peril, there is impending danger, or they are confronted with disaster. Even in the face of clear evidence and overwhelming proof to the contrary, people will continue expecting everything to continue to be OK or return to normal. A disaster warning that harm is about to displace what was their familiar and comfortable existence is interpreted and inaccurately reframed as nonserious with an expected positive outcome.

Why we continue to behave the way we do when the outcomes are so apparently going to be unpleasant is complex. But normalcy bias certainly appears to be a huge factor of the behavior. It's similar to the boiling frog metaphor. The story posits that if you put a frog in a pot of boiling water, it will instantly jump out. But if you put the frog in a pot of cold water and slowly turn up the heat, the frog will not do anything to improve its condition and eventually boil to death. The moral to the story is that people do not notice or respond appropriately to incremental change going on around them, or even clear and present danger, until it is too late.

Like with the Florida hurricane example, story after story exists of people who sit frozen rather than running or taking cover during tornados, terrorist attacks, or when they have only moments to remove themselves from a disastrous situation, such as from a plane or car after an accident. Experts believe such people need to be jolted, yelled at, smacked, or otherwise shocked into waking up and jumping out of the pot that's about to boil so they can save themselves.

The impending danger is quite clear.

We tend to think, "That won't be me." Rather, we imagine that in an emergency we'll be like the hero in an action movie and respond quickly, valiantly, abruptly, and save not only our own life but also the lives of those around us. But if you aren't living a life of wellness now, then you're the person sticking around to hang out during the hurricane. You're the frog in the pot. There's an urgent need for you to wake up!

Even still, there's hope. The reality is, you *can* be the hero and save yourself and the others who count on you. But you have to wake up and smell the coffee so you don't end up smelling boiled frog!

YOUR VALUE

An obvious rationale for not taking care of yourself would be somehow feeling that you aren't really worth it. You may look at your car, bank account, house, physical appearance, or occupation and decide that you are not as important as a neighbor, YouTube star, boss, or co-worker. The quick self-esteem assessment that follows will help you determine what you think of your value and inherent capability. It rates the overall positive or negative evaluation you have of yourself.

Strongly Disagree	Disagree	Agree	Strongly Agree
0	1	2	3

1. At times I think I am no good at all. _____

2. I take a positive view of myself. _____

3. All in all, I am inclined to feel that I am a failure. _____

4. I wish I could have more respect for myself _____

5. I certainly feel useless at times. _____

6. I feel that I am a person of worth, at least on an equal plane with others. _____

7. On the whole, I am satisfied with myself. _____

8. I feel I do not have much to be proud of. _____

9. I feel that I have a number of good qualities. _____

10. I am able to do things as well as most other people. _____

To determine your score, first reverse the scoring for the five negatively worded items (1, 3, 4, 5, & 8) as follows: 0 = 3, 1 = 2, 2 = 1, 3 = 0. Then add up your scores across the 10 items. Your total score should fall between 0 and 30. Higher numbers indicate higher self-esteem. —*Rosenberg self-esteem scale*

Your enduring self-esteem across time is known as your "trait self-esteem." Those who report high trait self-esteem now have high self-esteem later. Those with poor self-esteem early on tend to also have poor later.

"State self-esteem" is more changeable and reflects alterations in feelings and emotions. What you feel about yourself (your self-worth) and not your net worth is important. Otherwise, why invest in yourself? Unfortunately, people often tie their self-worth to their successes. Yet you are worth everything just as you are. The world may measure you by your measurements, but the world has it wrong.

When Jesus was baptized, God said of Him: "This is my beloved Son, with whom I am well pleased" (Matt. 3:17, ESV). This was before His ministry, before He turned water into wine, before He cleansed the lepers and raised anyone from the dead—including Himself. God lets us know that He loves Jesus because He is His Son and for no other reason. He loves the essence of Jesus as His child and a living, breathing human being.

God loves you in the same manner. Not because of your athletic prowess, appearance, bank account, car, title, education, house, relationship status, or even good deeds. He loves you like the most loving parent in the universe would love their child—with unmerited grace, immeasurable passion, and unlimited compassion. He loves you at and to the core!

YOU MATTER (YES, YOU)

Whether it seems like it or not, you matter. You matter to God, you matter to history, you matter to the world, you matter to the purpose you were created to serve, and you're needed by the people around you. You have tremendous value. Yes, you! Your value or worth is not determined by image.

In a world full of pain, confusion, and aimless materialism, your occupation, your finances, and your possessions might determine your position or image, but they have nothing to do with your worth.

As you aren't a measure of your successes, you aren't a measure of your struggles either. Once you've labeled yourself, you devalue yourself. If you call yourself poor, short, fat, ugly, divorced, addicted, lazy, a procrastinator, not a morning person, not an achiever, not a reader, a poor leader, old, arthritic, nonenergetic, and so on and on and on, then you start buying into and creating a destiny for which you weren't designed. Labeling has caused people to feel ashamed, defeated, and inadequate because they've been judged. They actually program themselves—or allow themselves to be programmed by those around them—to think of themselves as bad, unacceptable, abnormal, and less capable than all the other people on the planet.

This low self-esteem, poor-self-image mind-set that marks you as "unworthy" is faulty programming. But you can change all that—starting today. That's the great thing about life. It is not about the past; it's about the present and the future. In fact, the past has nothing to do with what you can do today or what you can accomplish tomorrow and for the remainder of your "tomorrows."

There's No "Bottom Line" Total for Your Worth

Your worth can't be counted in power, fame, fortune, or what you did or didn't do yesterday. It's based solely on the value of your uniqueness and all of your incredible potential. When a baby is born, it holds no job and has no possessions, yet its value is indescribable and its potential limitless. And here's the great part that most people don't realize: That value and potential you were born with don't leave or depreciate as you age! Isn't that awesome?

Think about it. Nothing is more common than people who seemingly have everything, yet because they've put their value in those things they lose sight of their worth and therefore who they are. Every year we see rich, beautiful, A-list celebrities face tragedies based on how miserable or lonely their lives have become. From our *perspective* they are on top of the world. But from their perspective, life is not worth living.

On the other hand, many clergy, teachers, civic servants, charity workers, missionaries, and others who serve those around them—though they have very little in the way of fame, money, power, or possessions—feel a deep sense of value and live incredibly fulfilling lives. What they don't accumulate in cash and the social-image bank account, they make up for with their investment in self-worth.

VISION

Visions are born in the soul of a man or a woman who is consumed with the tension between what is and what could be. Anyone who is emotionally involved, frustrated, brokenhearted, or maybe even angry about the way things are in light of the way they believe things could be is a candidate for a vision. Visions form in the hearts of those who are dissatisfied with the status quo.

chapter 4

WINNING THE INSIDE BATTLE

HAVE YOU EVER TAKEN A personality profile? Studies show they are extremely valid. One of the more common and accurate is the DISC profile. Most people who take it have to admit, it has them knocked. DISC stands for:

- D = Dominance: These are driven, Type A personalities.

- I = Influence: These are outgoing people who want to be liked.

- S = Steadiness: This personality is great for a loyal, supportive employee, friend, and spouse.

- C = Conscientiousness: This is the detailed, organized personality of the accountant, office manager, computer programmer, or math professor.

The first time I took it, I was all *D* and none of the other letters. It may be hard to imagine, but as a result I was single, with many bad relationships, and because I owned businesses and had no *C*, I suffered from several organizational train wrecks and lagged behind in technology. The DISC behavior model as proposed by William Moulton Marston, Ph.D., from Harvard in his 1928 book *Emotions of Normal People was to help people not only to understand their emotional behaviors, but also to measurably change these behaviors through their understanding.*

Unhappy with my catastrophic relationships and the continual fires I had to put out in my businesses, I took a hard look at my DISC personality. While it was far from easy at first, I had to pay attention to my lack of attention. I would need to be attentive to the needs and feelings of others like a functioning S would. Being unwilling to become a techie C person in today's technology-driven world is a horrible strategy. So despite all emotions to the contrary, I became passionate about details.

I still tend to want to outsource details and technology to others and can sometimes walk into work without saying, "Hi," but I talk back to my high D, my low S, and my low C, catch myself, and keep changing. Talking back against the parts of the profile you know you want to change and encouraging the one you want to rise up will help to rewire, reconstruct, and reshape your future.

What we've known since Marston close to a century ago is that over time we can make changes to our personalities. As you work toward the shift, realize that the old you still lives. The reality of the DISC is that for a time, your personality keeps crying out. Yet, I know thousands of formerly overweight, sleep-in people who are now very successful, up-early, fit people.

COGNITIVE DISSONANCE: OUR INNER CONFLICTS!

Pioneer researchers Leon Festinger and James Cardsmith discovered that there has to be a match between our thinking and our behaving. If not, our minds have to make adjustments to create consistency. If you think you should treat people better and drink less Mountain Dew, but you keep being mean to your co-workers and drinking that green chemistry experiment, then you have created a cognitive battle, or what Festinger and Cardsmith termed, "cognitive dissonance."[1]

Two dissonant positions create a real problem for you that your mind has to correct. The resulting stress of this inner conflict will move you to either align your beliefs with your actions or alter the belief.

Unfortunately, to release the pressure, you are most likely to take the path of least resistance by convincing yourself it is not important. You're also likely, then, to set up biases to keep it unimportant. Why? It is easier to stick to current wiring, reaffirm your biases, and continue down the road you're used to traveling. Consequently, in the mean co-worker/Mountain Dew case just mentioned, you can convince yourself that your co-workers deserve it and lean on your biases by deciding that the caffeine, sugar, and green dye aren't really harmful to your health.

You may wonder how people justify certain behavior that inflicts harm on themselves and those around them. The answer's pretty simple: It's because making the positive change is more difficult.

Sadly, however, *the soul knows*. Subconsciously, and often on a conscious level, the dissonance continues. You always lack real satisfaction until the best beliefs line up with the best practices for your future. This is the road "less traveled by…that has made all the difference."[2]

DISSONANCE AND THE FAILURE OF DIET PROGRAMS

Through my books *Body by God*, *Winning My Race*, the *Genesis Factor* and associated curriculum, I have conducted programs in thousands of churches around the world. The work is available in many languages. Yet, there is a church in my own city that wants nothing to do with wellness. While the biblical theme, "It's hard to be a prophet in your own town," may be at play here, so is cognitive dissonance. The pastor of this particular church weighs 300 pounds, smokes cigars, and drinks cognac. None of his lifestyle choices are my business, other than I wanted to help him and/or his church with their health.

Because of my family background, I have a unique level of love and compassion for people who struggle with their weight, and I offered to personally help him or anyone else since his church was right around the corner from my house. While he seemed very well-meaning, he was completely closed down to the idea. Instead, he drilled me on my knowledge of the Holy Trinity and remarked that lifestyle holds no value for the church. There was literally an oral exam on theology with no multiple choice. He told me I passed, but I believe he was just being nice.

This pastor clearly struggles with his lifestyle choices. If he allowed a wellness program to be launched at his church or even got help himself, he would be confronted with the fact that his choices do not line up with the recommended action.

This gets to one of the major reasons that diet books fail. To take on the full gospel of a diet plan, low-carb, no-carb, low-calorie, South Beach, Muscle Beach, The All Kale Plan—whatever—is to set yourself up for a moment of extreme dissonance. You are force-fed knowledge about why you must eat one way while old habits and the path of least resistance are leading you another. Eventually, the only way you'll survive is to get out.

What the pastor did not realize is that there are tricks to improvement that allow for incremental, permanent change that I would have guided him through. In fact, simple baby steps are proven to work, far more than quantum leaps are. It doesn't make sense to set someone up for failure and inner conflict. Rather than exploring the options, dissonance led this pastor to write off his health and that of his congregants entirely.

BECOMING UNCONFLICTED

Here are the steps for becoming *Just* unconflicted:

- Just say it – *Affirmations*
- Just do it – *Act as if*
- Just find a reason – *A why that makes you cry*

Just Say It—Affirmations

Festinger and Cardsmith were able to show that when someone speaks in favor of a viewpoint they don't agree with, their actual beliefs and opinions will begin to shift toward that viewpoint. This shift in thinking works more for those who actively communicate the differing belief than for those who just read about it or listen to information about it.

This means that even if you hate exercising, you will change your mind by talking about, reading about, and practicing exercise. The actions you take to reduce the dissonance will make you more likely to change your behavior so that it agrees with your new mind-set.

This discovery is the power of the spoken word. It's called "affirmations." Here's how they work for reconstructing purposes:

Saturday Night Live cast member Al Franken used to do a skit in which he hosted a one-on-one TV talk-show called *Daily Affirmations*. Before his guest came out, he'd look into a mirror and verbalize his affirmations. He'd say to himself: "I'm Good Enough; I'm Smart Enough; and Doggone-It, People Like Me!" The way he did it was funny, of course, but self-affirmation theory actually is an important concept that you need to add to your life. It is the idea that people can change thought processes, restore or maintain an overall sense of self-worth, and begin new behaviors that align with these new thoughts—despite beliefs or feedback to the contrary. Old thoughts and habits, insults, mistakes, failures, and rejection from others can throw us off course—but affirmations are there to course-correct us and keep us rewiring and refiring.

Affirmations Instructions

Step 1: What words describe what you want to start moving toward? Example: liking to exercise, enjoying natural foods, going to sleep before 11 p.m., waking up before 6 a.m.

Step 2: Based on what you want, what adjustments have to take place in self-talk?

Step 3: Rules for creating successful affirmations:

1. Start with the present: "Right now I am..."; "Every day I..."; "I'm regularly and continuously...."

2. Use emotion words: Enthusiastically, Excited, Energetically, Great rewards.

3. While reconstructing your thinking is a process that occurs over time, expect immediate results because soon results *will be* what you experience.

4. Read them daily: Put your affirmations on your bathroom mirror, in your car, at your desk, or anywhere else you will be sure to see them and recite them.

Examples of Successful Affirmations:_

*   Every day I am loving the feeling of exercise and getting leaner and stronger from my workouts!

*   Because of the nutrients I am putting in my body and the workouts I love, I am totally energized and able to come home and enthusiastically play games with my kids for hours!

*   I love the process of picking out and cooking fresh foods. These natural, health foods that are fresh instead of fast-food or microwaved taste amazing, are fun to make, and have brought my health and the way I look to another level!

Pay Attention to Reverse Affirmations and Eliminate Them:

- For example, here are some reverse affirmations that Al Franken's *Saturday Night Live* character could have said: "I don't know what I'm doing"; "They're going to cancel my show"; "I'm going to die homeless and penniless and twenty pounds overweight, and no one will ever love me." Don't use those.

French philosopher Voltaire once said: "No problem can withstand the assault of sustained thinking."

Affirmation Application—Do You Have Beliefs That Limit You?

Ask yourself these questions and answer them honestly:

- Have you ever started a diet on Monday and quit by Tuesday?
- Have you ever signed up for a gym membership, worked out for a few weeks, and then stopped?
- Have you ever bought a book, started reading it, and now you don't even know where that book is?
- Have you ever tried to lose weight and just quit because it wasn't happening fast enough?
- Do you believe that you are too old to lose weight?
- Do you believe that you will be on medications forever?
- Do you believe that because your mom is overweight that you will be too?
- Do you believe that you can't afford to eat well?

- Do you believe that your spouse will never change?

- Do you believe you can't change or overcome your circumstances?

If you said yes to any of these questions, then you have a "limiting belief." A limiting belief is one you have formed in your mind that is stopping you from making progress. You may be asking, "How do I know if I have any limiting beliefs?" The clue that you have a belief holding you back is the simple fact that you are not making any sustained progress in areas of your life that are important to you. It could be your weight, health, finances, relationships, work, and so on.

For example, let's say you set a goal to lose twenty-five pounds, so you start eating better and exercising every day. In only a few weeks you step on the scale and you've lost five pounds, you look better in the mirror, and everyone begins to notice your changes! Yet, soon you start skipping exercise, eating more desserts, and your new clothes stop fitting well. Rather than getting back to work, you ask yourself, "Why is this happening?" Or you say, "Here we go again."

Action step: Create affirmations that reverse these thoughts and open you up to thinking with no limits and unlimited possibilities.

JUST DO IT—ACT AS IF

"We are what we repeatedly do. Excellence, then, is not an act but a habit." —Aristotle

Traditional myths declare that genetics, in-born personality traits, and psychological characteristics determine how we act. Therefore, good people help old ladies cross the street, charismatic people become cheerleaders or politicians, and some people just happen to like sea lions. We have established, on the other hand, that you can change your way of thinking and thus your way of being.

I referred earlier to Ryle's, "The ghost in the machine." He was referring to our abstract mind controlling the path of material body, and not vice versa. Trees do not move the wind; the wind moves the trees—just as it is your spirit that's in control of your flesh and not your flesh that's in control of you!

Social psychologist and Cornell professor Daryl Bem said that when we take action toward the beliefs and personality we want to embody, we anchor to them.[3] Bem said:

- When we help someone in need to cross the street, it actually increases our desire to do good.

- As we lead people, it tells us we're charismatic motivators.

- When we enjoy the sea lions at the zoo, we assume we are lovers of sea animals.

This can be a negative or a positive in your life—it's your choice. For example, studies have revealed that taking sexual risks progressively increases risk-taking along with the associated pitfalls. Science reveals that people act in a way that is made more certain by action.

Bem's work, called "self-perception theory," has many positive uses for encouraging people to grow and take affirmative action to improve their lives. Rather than waiting for a magic moment when behavior will change, if you take action, attitudes and beliefs will follow. As taken from the words of

Aristotle, *"We are what we repeatedly do.* Excellence, then, is not an act but a habit."

Whereas the first action step to changing your thinking was saying, the next step is doing. As you start to act on the behaviors you desire, your thoughts and feelings about them have to follow suit. If you don't desire it or feel motivated to do it right now, the best way to change your thinking about it (according to another psychologist, Dr. Nike) is to: "Just do it!"

JUST FIND A REASON–A WHY THAT MAKES YOU CRY

People are motivated by a power higher than themselves and a purpose greater than theirs.

According to German philosopher Friedrich *Nietzsche,* "He who has a why to live *can* bear almost *any how."* Creating a powerful why, or a *why that makes you cry,* is another big step in the rewiring process.

As I mentioned, my dad died of a heart attack at the age of fifty-two. He allowed that daily grind that dads get into—to earn a living and manage family life—to cause him to ignore his body's limitations and, as a result, died before his time. Leading a life that way is done with the best of intentions, but it's really a crazy way to go. As parents push and drive to support their families and buy Christmas presents, they forget that more than anything, kids want their parents alive. I'd give up every present I ever received and would have gladly grown up in a box for the chance to see my dad even one more day.

My BIG WHY That Makes Me Cry

Death is rough at any point or any age for the people around you who care. Early death has the most severe collateral damage because it feels unjust. You feel like you've been ripped off.

The untimely demise of my father sent a painful shock wave through our family that we've not recovered from more than twenty years later. I wept enough for two lifetimes. After I had a family, I reflected on the unnecessary pain my mother, brothers, and I suffered and thought, *I don't want to leave my kids and my wife early if I can help it.*

While we cannot fully control our departure from this earth, I want my family to know I'm doing my part to stay! They are the reason why I try. They are my BIG WHY. The good of my family is what helps me stay focused on consistently making personal choices that support my being not just alive but also truly well for them.

I'm named after my grandfather, whom I never met. And my kids never met my dad. So often, being here for my family and the hope of being the first granddad in a couple of generations to meet the grandkids is how I overcome the temptation of addictions, don't give in to cravings, and overcome laziness. The *why that makes me cry* has wired me to exercise, eat well, and take my vitamins even when I don't want to do any of that.

"The mind is its own place,
and in itself can make a Heaven out of Hell
or a hell out of Heaven." —John Milton

Constructing Your Why

What is the most compelling reason for you to take control of your health? If you want to lose weight just to look good for the beach or a wedding, then that is not a why that makes you cry. Those are seasonal, temporary goals, and they don't rewire you, so they rarely work. When they do, it is generally not for very long.

Think about it: *What is your why that makes you cry?* Do you:

- Want to be there for your family?
- Wish to serve God in an extraordinary way?
- Want to walk or jog hand in hand with your spouse down the beach when you're past your 70s?
- See your grandchildren graduate and pass your wisdom on to them?
- Hope to avoid the early death or struggle with chronic disease your parents and relatives suffered from?
- Want to be a model of health for your family?
- Hope to advance your career?
- Want to experience longevity?
- Want to enjoy life to the fullest—finally?
- Hope to be independent and not become dependent on Depends (adult diapers)?

What Big Why or Whys are going to really move you and rewire you? This commitment to your cause or your purpose is another great motivator. People report better resolve, stronger will, and more sustainable discipline when working for a purpose bigger and greater then themselves. Some days, we just need a big reason to get out of bed. Health comes down to all of these little moments like the 2 minutes and 45 seconds of hell I discussed earlier. Getting up to exercise when the alarm goes off in the morning; having to dislodge yourself from the couch, desk chair, or car; purchasing or making the right food choice; passing on dessert and saying, "Just the check, please"; choosing the chicken or steak over the Fettuccini Alfredo—all these small moments of truth can be overcome by your Big Whys most of the time.

Affirm, Act, Why (AAW) Action Plan

Write down your affirmations, action steps, and Big Why or Whys on 3 x 5 cards so you can refer to them every day for the next thirty days. This will help to rewire your brain and reconstruct your thoughts x 30 and will jumpstart the process of authentic, long-term change.

HOW ABOUT A COMEBACK THIS YEAR?

I'm a sucker for a Cinderella story. I've got the original *Rocky* movie poster hanging in front of my treadmill at home. I love it because of the saying, "His whole life was a million-to-one shot."

Did you ever feel like that? Like all the odds have been or still are against you? Maybe, as a kid, it was the family you came from. Maybe you were short, unpopular, not athletic, had trouble with school. Or, as an adult, maybe you've lost money; blown relationships; become overweight; gotten depressed; developed joint pains; feel constantly fatigued, stressed, or overwhelmed; just not made the money or the impact on the world you once hoped you would. And on it goes.

What makes Rocky Balboa, James Braddock ("Cinderella Man"), the 1980 U.S. Olympic Hockey Team, Seabiscuit, *Pretty Woman*, and *Cinderella* such amazing stories is that, for them all, it was *over*. They were nothing, *nada*, already-blew-it, screwed-up, big-loser, forget-about-it, no-chance types. Yet, against all odds—when every normal, everyday motivation to keep trying would have run out or totally given up—theirs didn't. They did it, they made it. These so-called bums and losers *won*.

Do you remember a time when you wanted to do something significant, maybe even something great? What happened to that guy/girl? He or she existed once. Existed somewhere, long before there were the fears of failure, the mistakes, the goals you didn't hit when you wanted to hit them, bills to pay, and large-scale rejection. He or she existed long before these fears, pains, and frustrations caused you to justify your position or the position of others, turn excuses into reality, become a victim, and develop a deep fascination with self-preservation.

You Could Be the Next Rocky or Cinderella Story

How about a coming back to believing in yourself, knowing you're at cause and not a victim, believing in the fact that God did and still does have greatness and victory in store for you.

Could you be the Rocky or the Cinderella story of your town? The next miracle to shock the world? Absolutely! But, you have to know that you can do it, or at the very least be willing to try. Rocky said, "If I can go that distance, you see, and that bell rings and I'm still standin', I'm gonna know for the first time in my life, that I weren't just another bum from the neighborhood." He didn't know if he could do it, but he was willing to go for it. Once there, he called on all his past pain, all his unmet desires, and all his hopelessness and, rather than letting those emotions block him as they had in the past, he used them to find newfound hope, deep energy, and the will to go the distance.

What could you do? Abraham Lincoln's mother said to him from her deathbed: "Be somebody." What does "going the distance" mean in your life? What behemoth do you have to knock out or endure blow after blow from in order to be a champion in your own heart and the hearts of many? What do you have to do to be able to shout like Rocky, "Yo, Adrian, *I did it!*"

It's not the size of the dog in a fight, but the size of the fight in the dog. Fight comes from not quitting when things have been tough or failures have piled up over years and years. Fight comes when you use calamity and distress as inner fuel and failure as the very thing that propels you forward—or at the very least, to take the next step. No Cinderella story has ever happened because of great skills or natural ability. In fact, you *can't be* a Cinderella story unless you're a million-to-one shot! It's never been brains, arms, or legs that have won a place in history. It's been heart.

Rocky, James Braddock, the 1980 U.S. Olympic Hockey Team, and Seabiscuit (all true-ish stories), didn't really beat their opponents. They beat fear, frustration, desperation, and all that comes from a life that's said very clearly over and over and over again, "*You can't!*" Each, in their own way, conquered their own souls, and so can you!

Don't you think it's about time for a comeback? The entirety of Chapter 6 is dedicated to strategies and "Tricks" to make getting in good shape, even in great shape, easier for you to do than it is right now. It's dedicated to giving you everything you need to take your shot.

chapter 5

"THE BAD LIFESTYLE" PSA

One ship sails East,
And another West,
By the self-same winds that blow,
Tis the set of the sails
And not the gales,
That tells the way we go.

Like the winds of the sea
Are the waves of time,
As we journey along through life,
Tis the set of the soul,
That determines the goal,
And not the calm or the strife.

—ELLA WHEELER WILCOX

ARE YOU OLD ENOUGH TO remember those old-school PSA films on smoking and drunken driving? You know, the graphic ones? When I was growing up, they'd show them to us in school in hopes that we'd be "scared straight" and shun decisions to smoke or drink in excess. I still remember the side-effects-of-smoking pictures of black lungs; the interview with the 60-pound, bald woman with lung cancer; and the man talking through an electrolarynx after cigarettes gave him cancer of the larynx. The images are still etched in my head of mangled cars in deadly wrecks caused by drunk drivers; followed by images of the distraught moms and dads attending their teenagers' funerals.

If any of that's *too* old school for you, then you might not even know the term "PSA." It's short for "public service announcement." This chapter is my version of a PSA—"The Bad Lifestyle" PSA. It's a compilation of some facts about poor lifestyle and its effects on health that might just scare you straight. I considered not even including this chapter in the book, but I decided I wouldn't be fulfilling my obligation to humanity if I skipped it!

When I work with patients or clients who struggle to maintain a healthy lifestyle—who are overweight; frustrated; regularly eat, drink, or breathe in substances known to be bad for them; and who are experiencing unpleasant outcomes as a result, I become instantly super-curious. Every person who suffers in this way is someone I want to help. Plus, their insights and answers about why they struggle are learning pieces in a wellness-commitment puzzle that desperately needs to be solved.

SCARED HEALTHY

The numbers, as you'll see, do not lie: virtually every symptom and every disease is either mostly or completely caused by a hole in someone's lifestyle game. The bulk of our physical suffering, emotional crises, and displeasure with our appearance is self-induced. We are causing our own problems!

With these facts in mind, and coming from a very loving, sincere, and concerned place, I'll ask people with bad habits: "If you know these things are bad for you, how can you":

- Smoke?
- Eat a doughnut for breakfast?
- Drink alcohol nightly?
- Consume a soda every day or even worse, consume a diet soda every day?
- Never exercise?
- Consistently drop prescription or over-the-counter medications?
- Let you posture deteriorate like that?
- Stay up late when you have to be up early?
- (Feel free to add your own bad habit to the list!)

The answers I'm given are almost as varied as the habits:

- There are those who say they're ignorant of the facts.
- Others, I determine, are in denial.
- Some need a constant reminder to counter the habit
- Often they will tell me that, despite the evidence, they're just not convinced it's really causing them a problem.
- Or my least favorite: "I'm not hurting anyone."
- For most, they too are frustrated and want to stop but just can't fully motivate or commit themselves.

Many self-help books talk about a man, real or mythical, who came to his counselor for help because he wanted to stop smoking. As the story goes, he couldn't quit, did not really want to quit, and was seeking help only because his young family made him.

The counselor then asks him to imagine his daughter's high school graduation. Her hair and make-up are perfect, the ceremony is beautiful, there is an excitement in the air over students being released to take life to the next level, and his daughter glows as she glides across the stage to receive her well-earned diploma.

Afterward, she goes to greet the family. Everyone is hugging, congratulating her, and getting ready for the celebratory meal. But no one is smiling. Instead, there are tears. They are wishing Dad could have been there. But Dad died several years before from lung cancer.

Of course, in the storybooks, Dad is scared straight by picturing that scenario. He never smokes again. But the storybook version can be the real-life version too. A bad habit can be stopped cold in its tracks. That's a concept I supported in Chapter 4 when I discussed affirmations and the "Why that makes you cry" emotion.

Getting "scared straight" is a motivator that works immediately for some; for others, it's part of the process of waking up and starting to improve. I'll touch on some PSA points here, but I encourage you to use Dr. Google every chance you get to research them further. As you do you'll find that any symptom or illness you or someone you know suffers from has a lifestyle cause. Genetics makes up a very, very small percentage of the causes for conditions; and even when it is a contributor, it generally is your lifestyle that triggers the genetic involvement.

Why is that so important? Because you can start this journey to winning the inside battle as a *journey of hope*. You're not obligated to an unhealthy habit. You're not required to be a victim. There is hope when you know that for better or for worse you are responsible, all of us are the captains of our own ships, and for the most part it's we who determine which direction we go.

GENETICS

Conventional, traditional, outdated science would have us believe the reason our bodies are doing so poorly and, additionally, why we become rich or poor, happy or sad, addicted, overweight, disciplined or a procrastinator, healthy or diseased is as a result of genetics.

But the truth is: *DNA is not destiny.*

Your lifestyle is not based on some mere cosmic roll of the dice or some cruel or unfortunate genetic hand you may have been dealt. Attitude, body type, habits, health, as well as how our genes are expressed, are largely choices we get to make.

Your body is always naturally working toward homeostasis in order to stay well and constantly heal constantly. You might be asking, "Well if that's true, then why do so many people blame genetics for disease or other health issues?"

The Truth About Your Genes

This reason is the "gene myth." According to the newest research, dead relatives are not responsible for your health! It may surprise you to know the concept that "genes determine fate" has been disproved outside of an extremely small fraction of people.

The traditional field of genomics (the study of genes and their functions) has recently given rise to the more advanced science of "epigenetics." *Epi-* means "above or beyond." What you do, how you think, the way you behave, and the environment you live in are more powerful than your DNA and can turn off bad genes and turn on good ones—or vice versa.

It's true of course that genes and the DNA they're composed of are involved in carrying traits through generations. But genes alone are not responsible for the actual level of health you'll experience. Your DNA may write out the code for possible cell behavior, but those possibilities are realized only if the gene is expressed. We all have genes that are expressed and lead to physical or mental traits. Other genes, however, may remain silent. The ones that stay dormant do not have the ability to affect your behavior, health, or wealth.

Overall, it's more accurate to say that because you probably perceive the world, handle relationships, and live a lifestyle similarly to the way your parents did, you express similar genes. As a result, there is an obvious tendency to develop the same physical conditions. Nonetheless, you have something to say about your future. It is time to start living in a better way by living the life you want and not the one you believe you inherited!

We have the ability to control which genes will be expressed and which will not. The way you are living will influence the expression of your genes and allow you literally to model or remodel the functions of your body as well as the characteristics of your personality.

Two large-scale clinical studies from Northwestern University School of Medicine actually confirmed that the most important facets of healthcare, such as the no. 1 killer cardiovascular disease, have far more to do with lifestyle than genetics.

The first study evaluated five lifestyle factors: smoking, weight, exercise, diet, and alcohol consumption. More than 2,000 people were recruited for this study. The results showed that healthy lifestyle choices such as not smoking, exercising regularly, and not consuming alcohol excessively dramatically lowered the risk of developing heart disease.

A really important aspect to understand is that the more of these lifestyle essentials that were addressed, the lower the chance of disease. The risk only decreased by 6 percent for participants who changed just one lifestyle factor such as nutrition, but it decreased by 60 percent (10 times more) for those who made changes to all five lifestyle factors!

"Health behaviors can trump a lot of your genetics," said Donald Lloyd-Jones, M.D., chair and professor of preventive medicine at Northwestern University Feinberg School of Medicine and a staff cardiologist at Northwestern Memorial Hospital. "This research shows people have control over their heart health. The earlier they start making healthy choices, the more likely they are to maintain a low-risk profile for heart disease."

How does this happen? Genes load the gun, and environment pulls the trigger. We cannot change who are grandparents were or do anything about our genes. Thus, it makes absolutely no sense to worry about something you can do nothing about. The problem is, for many of us, if we do not change the direction of our lifestyle, we actually might end up where we are headed, and that is medication, surgery, or an early death. Your lifestyle does not get better by chance; it gets better by change, and you have the power to change it.

You may be defined, but you're not confined by your genetics—you have the final say in who, what, and how healthy you are!

PAUSE AND REFLECT

Our approach to health and health care just isn't working out—at all. People are entitled to their own opinions, but not their own facts. Here are the facts:

1. The amount of toxins in our environment, homes, food, and water are going up and up and up.

2. The amount of time we move and interact with other humans is going down and down and down.

3. We're taking more and more drugs.

4. We're getting sicker and sicker and adding new diseases into the mix regularly.

Snapshot of the Crisis:

- As many as 5 in 6 Americans die of heart disease and cancer.

- 4.5 million have Alzheimer's—a number that has doubled in the last two decades.[1]

- 118 million antidepressants are prescribed each year for some 57 million people with mental disorders.[2]

- 61 percent of American adults and 1 billion adults worldwide are overweight. The U.S. Congress calls this problem "as serious a threat as global warming."[3]

- In the last twenty years, the number of overweight children ages 6 to 11 has doubled—and tripled for adolescents.[4]

- More than 9 million U.S. children and 22 million children worldwide are diagnosed as being overweight and at risk of serious cardiovascular disease.[5]

- As weight is tied to conditions like high blood pressure, high cholesterol, and high blood sugar, these symptoms have raged out of control.[6]

- Conditions once set aside for adults only, such as adult-onset diabetes, high cholesterol, and high blood pressure, now impact millions of children as well.[7]

- Current mental health conditions are so bad that ordinary children are more fearful than psychiatric patients were in the 1950s.[8]

- Autism, a severe neurodevelopment disorder, impacts as many as 1 in 68 children, 1 in 35 if you're a boy (the conservative number is 1 in 110 children and 1 in 70 boys).[9]

- Circumstances have declined to the point that for the first time in history, this generation of children will experience shorter life expectancies than their parents.

The SAD Reality

The U.S. diet is called the Standard American Diet, or SAD.[10] These statistics show how sad it really is:

- 61 percent of American adults are overweight.
- 27 percent of Americans, or 50 million people, are obese.
- In the last twenty years, the number of overweight children between the ages of 6 and 11 have doubled.
- In the last twenty years, the number of overweight adolescents have tripled.
- Obesity doubles your risk of heart failure.
- Obesity raises breast cancer risks in women by up to 60 percent.
- A 15-pound weight gain in adults doubles the risk of developing Type 2 diabetes.

As reported in the *Wall Street Journal* article, "So Young and So Many Pills"[11]

- 1 in 4 children are taking chronic, lifetime drugs.
- 9 million are taking antidepressants.
- 6.5 million are taking antipsychotics.
- 5 million are taking blood pressure drugs.
- 300,000 are taking sleeping pills.

- 94,000 are taking statins (cholesterol-lowering drugs)

The lifestyle we follow and the environment we expose ourselves to are the combined cause of the crisis. While they can save a life in a crisis, the drugs we are turning to are not the answer; better living is.

YOU'RE LIVING IN A LIVING LABORATORY

Your body is an amazing, self-healing machine. Ponder for a moment the wonder and majesty of your body. You are made up of 50 trillion to 100 trillion cells. You create more than 100 billion new cells every day of your life. You get new lungs in sixty days, new skin in fourteen days, and a new heart in ninety days. You have an arsenal of white blood cells that identify and kill harmful invaders. Your red blood cells are amazing little vehicles that deliver oxygen to every nook and cranny of your body. Other cells carry electrical impulses that deliver important information to your brain. I could continue, but the point is clear: You are a walking, talking, self-healing miracle.

What does this mean for you? *If you supply your cells with the ingredients they need to function, they will work hard to keep you healthy.*

In order for you to have real health, the trillions of cells in your body need to create a balance of organ function, chemistry, and healing called "homeostasis." Excessive toxins and sugars, deficiency in nutrients, oxygen insufficiency due to a sedentary lifestyle, increased fat-to-muscle ratio, and continual emotional duress can individually cause harm—and be disastrous in concert.

In my eighth-grade science lab, we had to wear goggles any time we worked with chemicals or turned on a Bunsen burner. Why? Because chemicals are sensitive, and when you add or subtract new substances from the equation, something can explode. You're living in a laboratory called "the human body"—a living, experimental lab. In it, there's a continuous mass of volatile chemical reactions and equations occurring that must be handled with care. Like the science lab, your living lab is governed by organo-physical laws. Mess with those laws or poke that highly explosive bear and you'll not get a hall-pass from severe negative results. On the flip side, when you follow instructions and proceed as directed, the results are fun and interesting, and go more as planned.

THE E WORD

Exercise—it's an eight-letter word that has become twice as bad as a four-letter word! Nonetheless, your most important body parts, such as your heart, lungs, spinal column, muscles, veins, and arteries, require movement to function well. And in today's sedentary world, you have to create movement through planned exercise. For many people, exercise is like eating a rat sandwich—even anticipating it hurts, and it's hard to swallow. (If that's you, don't worry about it now; in the next chapter, I'm going to give you the many Tricks and secrets to successful exercise).

Most people have been taught to believe that if you're thinner or lighter it means you're healthier. But, the truth is, if you just starve yourself, follow some weird diet, take pills, or do bariatric surgery, you may lose weight, but you're just skinny sick or thin fat. The result: *you'll just die lighter.*

You become healthier only when your cardiovascular system (heart, lungs, and blood vessels) are dealing with oxygen (O_2) more efficiently and you have a good ratio of muscle mass vs. fat mass (loosely packed muscle). Being fit is vitally important to both physical and mental wholeness. Heart and lung function as well as optimal body composition (a high muscle-to-fat ratio) are critical survival needs and can't be improved through diets, pills, potions, drugs, surgery, or electric stimulation alone. No matter what the infomercial tells you, you'll have to actually *move!*

While traditional means of treating and preventing illnesses and improving poor physical test results have failed to give us much to rejoice about, exercise is consistent at providing huge health benefits. The *E* word will:

- Improve heart function
- Lower blood pressure
- Reduce body fat
- Elevate bone mass
- Decrease total and LDL cholesterol ("bad" cholesterol)
- Raise HDL cholesterol ("good" cholesterol")
- Raise energy level
- Enhance and balance hormone production
- Aid in the sleeping process
- Increase stress tolerance
- Eliminate toxins

- Reduce depression
- Control or prevent diabetes (blood-sugar issues)
- Decrease the risk of injury to the muscles, joints, and spine

Exercise, Oxygen and Lean Muscle

How much lean muscle compared to body fat you have matters for more than dress sizes and Speedos. Better lean-muscle-to-body-fat ratios play a big role in overall health.

Oxygen is a more important elemental nutrient for survival than any nutrient you can swallow. Oxygen has been shown to stymie the growth of cancers. Healthy cells love oxygen, and cancer cells hate it. It makes sense, doesn't it?

The far-too-sedentary American lifestyle represents one of the deadliest carcinogens out there. Our couch-potatoism leads to obesity, and extra fat leaves your body more susceptible to cancer. In addition, lack of exercise, no matter what your weight, still puts you at a higher risk for cancer.

Building muscle and losing fat diminishes your chances of developing cancer of any type. For example, a study of 13,000 men and women whose progress was followed for fifteen years by aerobics guru Dr. Kenneth Cooper showed that poor diet and lack of exercise caused as much as 60 percent of all colorectal cancers in men and 40 percent in women. Over all, out-of-shape people were shown to be 300 percent more likely to develop cancer.

Cancers directly linked to lack of exercise include those of the:

- Breast (among women who have gone through menopause)
- Colon and rectum
- Endometrium (lining of the uterus)
- Esophagus
- Kidney
- Pancreas

Being overweight may also raise the risk of these cancers:

- Breast
- Gallbladder
- Liver
- Non-Hodgkin's lymphoma
- Multiple myeloma
- Cervix
- Ovary
- Aggressive forms of prostate cancer

The powerful effect that a properly applied exercise program has on physiology is the key reason for its cancer-stopping effects. Exercise improves:

- Cardiovascular capacity
- Lung capacity
- Circulation
- Immune function, such as an increase in white blood cells, interleukin or neutrophils
- Speed and function of bowel motility

- Antioxidant defenses
- Ideal hormone levels

The right kind of physical training lowers bad hormone levels, increases good ones, boosts immune functions, helps manage weight, and lowers body fat. Each of these benefits counteracts known causes of breast cancer.

If exercise were a drug, it would be considered the miracle cure the world has been looking for since antiquity. Of course, the positive benefits of exercise all work in reverse if you are not active and you're unfit. Systems, hormone levels, oxygen efficiency, and cell and organ function all move toward an unhealthy or even disease state for those who aren't doing some form of physical training at a minimum of three days a week.

SUGAR: THE OTHER DEADLY WHITE POWDER

We've all heard about the addictive properties of cocaine. In its most common form, it's an innocuous-looking white powder that when used is addictive, ruins lives, and can have potentially deadly consequences. I call sugar "the other deadly white powder." While some people are more carb-tolerant than others, most of us are not. Even the people who seem to burn the sugar well for now normally pay a hormone price later. And it's everywhere: whether you put the white packet ingredients in your coffee, eat a Snickers bar, an apple, bread, rice, or pasta, the downline effect of carbohydrates is always sugar in your system.

In the process of taking in sugar, insulin (a hormone) is required for the cells to absorb it. At modest doses of slow-burning sugars this mechanism will serve you just fine, and for a long, long time. Excess energy is what creates a problem.

Excess sugar requires excess insulin. If you're continually eating carbs, eventually the presence of insulin in the system is ignored by the cells. Too many carbs cause the insulin to keep knocking on the door of the cells (called "receptors"). But the cells start to ignore the knock like it's a bad neighbor. Insulin keeps calling, and the cells just keep sending to voicemail. This situation is called *insulin resistance*, and it sets you up for series of unfortunate events:

- The excess sugar gets stored as fat
- The brain starts to become resistant to other fat and appetite-balancing hormones.
- Triglycerides and high bad cholesterol start to rise
- Inflammation, oxidation, and bad aging occur from all the sugar processing
- A litany of chronic diseases associated with the points just listed can occur.

In reality, getting fat is a metabolic marker that signals the presence of too much carb energy and the growing inability of your body to manage all the sugar and excess fat it creates. This is why we say, "Carbs kill."

Sugar Feeds Cancer

Like all causes of cancer, sugar interferes with normal, healthy, balanced physiology. What makes sugar even more of a problem is that cancer really thrives on it.

When a patient goes in for a PET (positron emission tomography) scan to see if cancer is spreading, he or she is administered dextrose, a form of sugar. Shortly before a PET scan is performed, the patient is injected with the dextrose, which also contains a radioactive dye. The cancer cells eat the sugar, and the dye illuminates the cancer-affected areas of the body.

High blood-sugar and insulin levels also lead to elevated levels of insulin-like growth factor-1 (IGF-1). Elevated IGF-1 plays a major role in the progression of many childhood cancers and in the growth of tumors in breast cancer, small-cell lung cancer, melanoma, and cancers of the pancreas and prostate, according to researchers at the National Institutes of Health. This has been confirmed many times.

Whether it's the insulin, the body fat, the inflammation, or the negative impact on hormones, many studies support the flat-out fact that sugar equals cancer. The *Journal of the National Cancer Institute* in 2004 showed that women who ate the highest glycemic (sugary) foods were three times more likely to develop colon cancer.

Sugar is a hidden danger in many foods. According to published reports, the top source of sugar for the vast majority of North Americans is soft drinks. Other sources include processed meats, pizza, sauces, breads, soups, crackers, fruit drinks, canned foods, yogurt, ketchup, and mayonnaise. Read the ingredients! You'll be shocked. This deadly white powder is consumed at an average of 120 pounds per person each year.

Our list of healthy carbs AND grain-free and sugar free-recipes, as well as our guide to killing the carbs will provide you with plenty of tricks for winning the battle against excessive carbs in your diet. (See Chapter 6)

FINAL SCENE IN "THE BAD LIFESTYLE" PSA

As I said, my goal with this chapter is to wake you up and make you aware, like those frightening "don't smoke" or "don't drink and drive" PSA movies were intended to do. Hopefully you have the visual: too much of the wrong food, too much sugar, or too little of the right exercise, and the scene gets gruesome and deadly—but, hopefully in your case, only memorable.

Of course, like the many kids who saw those movies and still smoked or got behind the wheel drunk, you might not be scared straight—or "scared thin"—by what you've just read. It's imperative, however, that you do not deny the facts. In my PSA "movie," when my mom reached for one cigarette after another, I do not believe she envisioned her children taking care of her like she was their child, as has been the case. When my dad said he'd rather be dead than eat "this way," he just did not believe there would ever be a scene showing his eighteen-year-old son Rich finding him on our front lawn and trying desperately and unsuccessfully to save his life when he was only fifty-two.

In 12-step recovery programs, most therapists will say that Step 8 is where the person's recovery often comes apart. In this step, the substance addict has to make a written list of all persons they have harmed along the way and be willing to make restitution to each one. Our choices impact people—like my little brother was impacted by finding and trying to save my dad or like our whole family was impacted by his death or my mother's habit-induced disability.

The sick, the unhealthy, or the addicts who have told me, "I'm not hurting anyone," have always been very, very wrong. In their cases, there were always specific individuals, if not dozens of loved ones around them. whose lives were stressed, wrecked, or totally ruined from dealing with the collateral damage of their lifestyles. These scenes and facts surrounding them aren't true just in the movies or for someone else; they are real for you and for the people around you.

There's only one way to change your story. Write a new script.

MAKING CHANGE WORK

I was taught early on that the reason people are often unable to start making positive change or they quit during the process even when they are experiencing great results is that they:

A. Get lost with no one to point them in the right direction

B. Have questions that need to be answered for them to continue

C. Get confused

D. Lose hope

Hopefully, you've learned quite a bit about your possibilities for change and success at this point, and you may even be more motivated after my PSA announcement. To make sure change is easy, at least easier, and that you do not fall victim to A-D on why people fail or quit, I have provided in the last chapter a final piece to the puzzle. These are the tools required to stop, enjoy, and complete any plan. In fact, most of what I do online or in my coaching programs is to just keep offering tools to make life fun and change easy while you get healthier and feel and look better and better. Put the tools to work, and build the future you want.

chapter 6

10 TRICKS FOR A CHANGE: HOW TO CHEAT THE SYSTEM

DECADES AGO, PSYCHOLOGIST WALTER MISCHEL, Ph.D., did a seminal study of self-control. In it, preschoolers were given a plate of kid treats such as marshmallows. The child was told the researcher was going to leave and that the child had a choice to make:

- If they could wait until the researcher came back, they could have double the marshmallows.

- If they could not wait, they would get just one marshmallow.

This was the consummate study in the ability to delay gratification and the self-control necessary to sacrifice immediate pleasure in lieu of a greater opportunity at a later point in time.[1]

TRICKING YOURSELF INTO A BETTER FUTURE

Our ability, then, to put off sleeping in this morning, the cigarette right now, the doughnut now so that we might experience success, better health, or the body we want later is a measure of self-control that can make all the difference in so many important areas of life. As the study shows, it can reveal information on areas like performance, emotional stability, relationships, and career down the road.

Mischel continued to track the success of children who participated in the marshmallow experiment. As teenagers, for example, those who had waited longer for the marshmallows as preschoolers were more likely to score higher on the SAT. Also, their parents were more likely to rate them as having a greater ability to plan, handle stress, respond to reason, exhibit self-control in frustrating situations, and concentrate without becoming distracted.[2]

The Marshmallow Test emphasizes the detrimental predilection toward "hyperbolic discounting." This refers to the tendency for people to choose a smaller-sooner reward over a larger-later reward. If this were money we were talking about, the result would be that you'd take $50 now rather than wait and get $100 next month. This inability to delay gratification, or lack of self-control, has implications in all areas, as the researchers found, not just in our dietary habits.

Researchers tracked down the study participants into their 40s and tested their willpower and self-control. Incredibly, their willpower differences held up. Generally, the kids who had been less able to resist eating the marshmallows all those years ago also performed more poorly on self-control tasks as adults.[3]

An interesting side-note: To investigate why some people seem inherently more capable of self-control than others, the researchers also examined brain activity in the marshmallow participants and found more activity in the executive center of the brain. This again is the prefrontal cortex, the part of the brain responsible for choices, addictions, and self-discipline.

Mischel states: "By harnessing the power of executive function and self-control strategies, we can all improve our ability to achieve our goals."

These kids learned to trick themselves into not eating the marshmallow. They looked away from it, tapped their fingers, counted, diverted their attention and hid their eyes from seeing what they wanted now to gain a better return in the future. Those are executive strategies—or "tricks," as I call them—these children used.

Adults need executive strategies, too. We need ways to trick ourselves into self-control for success in all areas of life. Along with the activities I have already shared, tricks, strategies, food lists, and healthful recipes make up the remainder of this book.

TRICKS AND STRATEGIES

1. The 4 Keys: Plan, Prepare, Cook & Shop
2. The Jack Lalanne Tenet
3. Overcome Weight Loss Resistance

4. The Food Change Rules

5. Carb and Protein Counter and List of Good fats

6. Seven-Day Diet Diary

7. Quick workouts with long impact

8. Executive strategies: Goal form, Diet diary, Reading food labels, and Time Management/Solid Yellow Line Sheet

9. Food list

10. Recipe and Snack suggestions

TRICK #1: THE 4 KEYS: PLAN, PREPARE, COOK & SHOP

Focus on the four keys to better eating. You may want to eat well; but if the wrong food is in the house, at work, in the car, on an airplane, and you have not planned to eat well, you will fail.

1. Plan

Know what you are going to eat for the day. Plan your menu for the whole *week*. When it comes to eating, the adage "Failing to plan is planning to fail" has never been more true.

2. Prepare

Make sure you have made or packed the food you will need order to eat better. For example, school and work lunches and snacks packed in the minicooler. If you get caught at school, work, or on the run without the right food, you'll end up eating the *wrong* food.

3. Cook

Good food is almost always *prepared, cooked,* or *plucked* and is rarely *ripped open* from a package where it is ready to eat.

Great tip: Try to cook for more than *one* meal at a time so that healthy, cooked, or prepared food becomes your "fastest food."

4. Shop

You cannot eat well if you have not bought the food you need. Make sure your kitchen is stocked with what you will need in order to lead a more nutritious life. The stuff at the back of the shelves in your pantry is rarely the *healthy stuff.*

TRICK #2: FOLLOW THE JACK LALANNE TENET: "IF GOD DIDN'T MAKE IT, DON'T EAT IT."

"Man-food" is food human beings create or alter. It is also food not intended for humans to use expressly on a regular basis. Avoid man-food.

Many types of man-food are recommended by different diets. These fad programs utilize unnatural foods and pre-packaged foods that contain processed animal products, chemical-containing powders and meal replacements, and certain stimulant supplements. They may produce weight loss short-term and in very rare cases even long-term. They don't, however, produce health. You won't make it long-term.

The farther you get from eating the foods specifically created for the body, or the farther these foods are from their natural form, the less efficiently the digestive system can break them down—if it can at all.

Jack Lalanne, a fitness guru that was still pulling tugboats with his teeth at 90 years old once said, "If God didn't make it, I won't eat it!" This is a great tenet to live by. If you do only one thing with your nutrition, at all, do this: *Go natural!*

TRICK #3: OVERCOME WEIGHT-LOSS RESISTANCE (WLR)

Our calorie consumption as a nation actually doesn't match up with our enormous, exponential rise in obesity. The "weighty" predicament we're in is, in reality, being created by the onslaught of refined, toxic foods; an excess of sugar and sugar-based preservatives in our diet; an enormously sedentary lifestyle; and, equally important, our stressed and rushed culture.

They have resulted in an assortment of "metabolic damage" factors that have created not only additional weight gain but also weight-loss resistance. These metabolic factors actually make it extremely difficult if not impossible to lose fat! This may explain in your case why you've tried but failed to lose weight.

For many people, just following Jack Lalanne and going all whole, God-made food will resolve their weight issues and even solve the weight-loss-resistance issues. By contrast, there is a segment of the population who has damaged their metabolism to the point of being severely weight-loss resistant. They must heal these areas before their bodies will really be able to burn fat and hold on to or build lean tissue.

Why Weight Loss Is So Important

The scientific community was recently shocked when the *New England Journal of Medicine* released several studies showing that even being moderately overweight and having no symptoms of poor health gives you as high as a 30 percent (1-in-3) mortality rate (chance of dying).[4]

In order for your body to lose weight, the hormones, insulin, and leptin must be doing their work. Remember, insulin is in place to control sugar and fat-storage levels in the body. Leptin's job is the burning of fat. If these hormones and the mechanisms that are there to utilize them aren't working, then you will be unable to lose weight and extremely prone to packing it on. Here are the three reasons these hormones begin to fail in your body:

- Too many sugars, processed grains, and whole grains
- Toxicity
- Exercise that ups good hormones rather than bringing them down

The ABCs of Overcoming WLR
A. Detox

When toxins enter your body, they have an affinity for fat cells and throw off some of the many hormone responses in your body that are involved with weight loss. When you are toxic, you can also feel horrible and cannot figure out why. You find yourself on medications, chasing symptoms on a never-ending downward spiral.

Detox Basics

Salads and raw vegetables contain the ingredients for your body to make its own detoxifying agent "glutathione." Therefore, minimizing exposure to household chemicals, medications, personal-care products, and artificial foods while maximizing a raw, whole-food diet with less grains and sugar supports the body's own inherent detox systems.

B. De-Stress, Get Some Rest, and Take B Vitamins

Important stress effects on your physique[5]:

1. Stress raises cortisol, the catabolic hormone that causes you to put on fat, lose muscle, resist insulin, want to eat more, and crave sugar.

2. Chronic stress lowers serotonin and makes you hypoglycemic—both of which cause you to crave sugar.

3. Chronic stress affects your body's ability to build muscle. Lean muscle is your "metabolic girdle," which is the key factor for metabolism.

4. Stress depletes B vitamins so that your body can't make the neurotransmitters needed to help you go to sleep and stay asleep.

5. Less sleep = elevated cortisol, less of the antiaging hormone melatonin, and less blood-sugar control.

   - People who sleep two to four hours a night are 73 percent more likely to be obese

   - Those who get five hours of sleep are 50 percent more likely to be obese.

- Those who sleep six hours are 23 percent more likely to be obese.

- Those who get 10 or more hours are 11 percent less likely to be obese.

The top causes of stress are not sleeping, rushing, caffeine, sugar, and continuous emotional turmoil. All play a role in causing too much tension and making it challenging if not impossible to lose weight and look good.

C. SURGE: Short-Duration, High-Intensity Exercise

Today people realize that being fit is a necessity to being healthy, preventing and overcoming disease, and protecting the spine and joints. Still, for most people, exercise remains more of a hated event, like the office Christmas party or wedding of a distant relative.

When surveyed, some common excuses people give for not exercising are: boredom, pain or injury, no place to do it, and can't afford it. But the megaexcuse that 75 percent give as the reason they don't exercise is: they don't have the *time*.

The good news is, there is now a method of exercise you can do in only twelve minutes a week without leaving your home or office. It's called Surge Training—and it's the new aerobics.

To understand the power of the Surge, you first have to abandon much of what you've been taught about exercise. Most of us have learned that what happens to you *during* exercise is what's important. But, in reality, what's more important is what happens *after* exercise. It's how your body responds that has the greatest impact on your physique and the many layers of your health.

The aerobic craze started back in the 1980s with Richard Simmons, disco music, and a whole lot of colorful spandex. Unfortunately, even today, people still associate exercise with that type of program. As a result, exercise has come to mean long periods of time on a treadmill or other piece of "cardio" equipment. And the longer the time, the better. Thus the excuse: "I don't have time."

This type of cardiovascular exercise is also known as 'low-intensity, long-duration" activity, and there are several physiological and hormonal problems related to this old, out-dated, so-called classic exercise concept.

The following are the pros and cons of classic aerobics. I'm sure you'll see why it's time to throw out the spandex, the 8-tracks, the Richard Simmons videos, and other related classics.

Effects of Long-Duration, Low-Intensity "Classic" Aerobic Exercise

Research done on both elite and novice athletes shows that the benefits of low-intensity, long-duration activity are far outweighed by the benefits of high-intensity, short-duration activity. What we call Surge Training.

Pros That Occur During Exercise

Lowers resting heart rate and increases stroke volume

- Lowers blood pressure
- Keeps brain young by increasing circulation to the brain
- Aids detoxification, stimulates the lymphatic system

Cons That Occur After Exercise

- Raises stress hormones: The stress hormone cortisol stimulates appetite, is catabolic (breaks down muscle), increases fat storing, and slows down or inhibits exercise recovery

- Decreases testosterone and Human Growth Hormone (HGH)—both necessary for building muscle and burning fat.

- Decreases immune function post-exercise

Therefore, while there are benefits to classic aerobic activity, the response you're left with is a broken-down, fat-storing, muscle-wasting state. This is why we hear our patients and readers complaining all the time that they've been exercising and exercising but just can't seem to lose any weight.

- The Powerful Effects of High-Intensity, Short-Duration Exercise HGH is released in the body in direct proportion to exercise intensity.

- There is a greater increase in fat expenditure after high-intensity exercise due to the HGH release.

- There is a positive relation between carbohydrate expenditure during intensive exercise and fat expenditure during recovery

- Muscle triglyceride lipolysis is stimulated only at higher exercise intensities.

- Beta-endorphin levels associated with positive changes in mood are increased in short-term intensity exercise. (Better than an antidepressant!)

119

- HGH, an activator of lipolysis and muscle growth, is stimulated by the exercise-intensity threshold.

- Plasma glutamine is decreased after long-duration exercise and increased after short-term, high-intensity exercise.

- Contribution of both type I and type II muscle fibers, and hence a decrease in age-related muscle atrophy.

With high-intensity, short-duration exercise your body *responds* by increasing the hormones and physiology you need to burn fat and produce muscle. As a result, your body not only builds muscle and burns fat *during* exercise, but it also responds by doing so for hours *after*.

Plus, the more muscle you have, the more tendency there is to produce more muscle. It's muscle and not age, gender, or genetics that is the greatest determining factor for metabolism and future muscle development.

Even better, if you can combine this with an aerobic effect, you'll get the benefits of classic aerobics without the negative side-effects. That's why we call this the "New Aerobics."

SURGE TRAINING
The New Aerobics: Fast, Fun, Effective, and No Spandex

Surge Training consists of intermittent bursts, or surges, of energy. It's similar to the concept of interval training, only it's done within a more limited time frame and with a strong focus on the importance of the recovery time.

The idea of the *surge* is to safely shock your body into responding physiologically so that you're left in a more ideal state metabolically for getting tone and getting into better condition. After a maximum energy output, the body must respond. After a Surge, it responds or adapts by altering hormones and physiology so that your body is burning fat and building muscle—during *and* after the exercise activity.

Anyone can do it, and it's safe. The reason it's safe is that your maximum output is what is right for you, individually. You can go at a maximum without using heavy weights or overstraining your joints or muscles. It's a superior workout that can be done by anyone, from a beginner trying to drop pounds to an Olympic or professional athlete trying to compete at the highest level.

Before Starting, Find Your Training Heart Rate With the Following Calculation:

1. 220 minus Your Age = Your Maximum Heart Rate

2. 75 percent to 85 percent of your Maximum Heart Rate is your Training Heart Rate. Add 10 to your Training Heart Rate if you're an experienced athlete. Subtract 10 if you're a beginner or experiencing or recovering from health problems.

NOTE: *Stop the workout if you're not an elite athlete and your heart rate reaches 100 percent or more of your Training Heart Rate. Always consult a physician before starting any new exercise program.*

In a Surge set, you do a maximal output for a minimum of 10-15 seconds and a maximum of 60 seconds. Only elite athletes have the capacity to keep a maximum output for 60 seconds. Then you recover just long enough to allow your heart rate to approximate normal or Resting Heart Rate and you surge again. Recovery time is usually equal to the effort time.

After the Surge, you'll find out why we also call this aerobics. *Aerobic* means to exercise "with air"—and you'll definitely be breathing more heavily and feeling your cardiovascular system getting a workout.

BASIC SURGE PROGRAM

Example: Surge Training using a stepper, stepping up and down on a step, or simply stepping up and down in place on the floor as fast as you can. (This can also be done while lifting a weight from your side up and over your head to add resistance into the movement):

1 SURGE:

20 SECONDS ON (Heart rate up to the Training Zone)

20 SECONDS OFF (Full recovery time to get heart rate back to the bottom of the Training Zone or below.)

20 SECONDS ON

20 SECOND OFF

20 SECONDS ON

2 MINUTES OFF (Recovery is important for full surge effect).

- *Repeat this cycle three or four times for 3-4 minutes of total exercise, or approximately 12-15 minutes total elapsed time.*

- Lower or increase the time based on your ability to sustain a maximal effort. You lose the shock effect once you begin to slow down. Recovery should equal the time of the surge. **The recovery time is incredibly important.**

- **Total exercise time for an entire week on the basic program is only 12-16 minutes, and total elapsed time for an entire week is an hour or less!*

- Who can use *time* as an excuse now for not getting healthy and in the shape of your life? What works better for your busy schedule? Three minutes a day of exercise or 24 hours of being dead?

- Endurance athletes can work this into their weekly trainings and/or increase the number of surges per session to radically improve their performance times.

Another Great Way to Surge

Pick 6 exercises that tax the system. Examples: push-up, overhead press, burpees, band curls, mountain climbers, plank.

- Do each exercise hard for 1 minute

- Rest 30 seconds

- Repeat

- Total elapsed time: 12 min./30 sec.

WEIGHT TRAINING WITH QUICK SETS

To get even faster changes in your body and overall health, add weight training on the days you're not Surging or right before your Surge.

The Quick Set program is the weight-lifting portion of the Surge program.

Quick Sets Give More for Less. In weight-resistance training, utilizing similar principles to Surge Training allows you to work an individual body part in as little as three minutes. Plus, these Quick Sets are radically more effective than typical, longer exercise sessions.

By performing Quick Sets, you are able to create significant changes in the composition (body-fat percentage and muscle tone) of a body part within three minutes. This will radically lower your BMI (body mass index). These routines can be used to increase the intensity of your workouts, shorten your workout times, and very safely speed up your results. They are designed so that anyone can perform them and make great changes on any level. Whether you are simply trying to lose the spare tire or pick up an Olympic medal, Quick Sets will work for you.

For the purpose of fitness, there are only eight body parts to consider: chest, biceps, triceps, shoulders, abdominals, back/lats, legs (which include quads, hams, glutes, inner/outer thighs), and calves. By exercising with squats or lunges, you can actually hit your hamstrings, quads, the glutes (butt), and inner and outer thighs (typical trouble spots for women) all with one exercise.

Hit each body part once per week, and you'll invest only about 24 minutes to get into great shape! Add that to the 36 minutes of cardiovascular Surge Training and you get maximum exercise benefits for a *total elapsed time of 60 minutes—one hour—per week!*

PERFORMING QUICK SETS
Decline Quick Set

1. Pick one exercise and do it for 8 to 12 repetitions until failure.

2. Rest for 5 or 6 seconds.

3. Lower the weight 5 to 20 pounds and do the same exercise again for 6 to 8 repetitions until failure.

4. Rest 5 or 6 seconds.

5. Lower the weight 5 to 20 pounds again and do another 6 to 8 repetitions until failure.

Pause Quick Set

1. Pick one exercise and do it for 8 to 12 repetitions until failure.

2. Rest 5 or 6 seconds.

3. Using the same weight, do the exercise again until failure.

4. Rest 5 or 6 seconds

5. Repeat this process until you cannot do the exercise for more than 1 or 2 repetitions.

Monster Set

A Monster Set is when, after performing an exercise on one body part, instead of resting, you immediately perform an exercise on *another* body part. The other body part should be one that was not used while exercising the first body part. For example, combine chest and biceps, or quadriceps and hamstrings.

Monster Sets are combined with Decline or Pause Sets so you can get a tremendously effective workout done in a very short amount of time. For example, after you perform a Pause Set with the incline fly press for your chest, you can immediately begin performing a Decline Set with hammer curls for your biceps.

With high-intensity, short-duration exercise your body *responds* by increasing the hormones and physiology you need to burn fat and produce muscle. As a result, your body not only builds muscle and burns fat *during* exercise, but also responds by doing so for hours *after*. *This may be the best trick there is!*

TRICK #4: THE FOOD CHANGE RULES

Due to growing up and watching my parents hate the food change they made, I became like a mad scientists developing formulas for how to make eating well easier.

When I originally began working with people to help them change their eating habits, the average person would fail miserably. The standard method of nutritional change is to take somebody's existing diet, throw it in the trash, and then hand them a completely new way of eating.

When I first started counseling, this method of "out with the old, in with the new" caused the average person who came to me for weight loss to gain four pounds per week while under my care. Even cancer and diabetes patients would not follow my diet. They would rather die. No one to whom I ever gave a totally new diet for any reason ever stuck to it for more than a few days or, in some cases, a few minutes.

Following and sticking to a brand-new way of eating is extremely hard. In some cases, it is impossible. That is why I created the Food Change Rules to help people get better at eating over time. As a result of these simple 6 Rules, I have achieved results with thousands of people who thought they would never be thin or healthy again or who had failed on numerous occasions to eat better.

1. The Addition Rule

The National Weight Control Registry has been tracking weight loss for over three decades and found what you would expect: that a very small amount of people can lose any substantial amount of weight or, if they do, maintain weight loss. Their investigation shows that dieters fail when attempting to eat many right foods all of the time. Those who succeeded, however, managed to make small, incremental forward progress like adding an apple to breakfast in the morning.[6] Not exactly the stuff of *New York Times* best sellers, but effective in proactively producing change.

Positive eating habits are best formed as a positive, gradual process and not an overwhelmingly negative process. To be effective and long-lasting, change must come slowly, so as not to shock the system or the brain.

The Addition Rule states that instead of eliminating the bad, you add the good.[7] So for those of you who drink diet soda and eat a candy bar for breakfast every morning—don't just stop that behavior and start eating nothing but fruit. If you do, you will only quit, or your brain will explode; whichever comes first.

What the Addition Rule has you do is add an apple to your cola and candy bar breakfast. With the Addition Rule, you do not take away, you *add*.

Most people are overfed but undernourished. There is no nourishment in their diet. Many modern diets literally contain no real food at all. It is all just fast food, junk food, quick food, and refined food, all of which are full of calories but devoid of nutrition. By adding healthy foods, you become not only fed but nourished as well.

The idea of elimination tends to create negative thought patterns in the brain. The feeding system responds better to positive patterns than to negative ones. Eliminating negative food items from an unhealthy diet is a much more challenging task than simply adding positive things to the diet a little at a time.

Therefore, begin thinking positively and not negatively. To do so, call on the first rule of nutrition, the Addition Rule. Adding an apple does not do much to eliminate the ill effects of consuming other unhealthy foods. However, it does add a significant level of nutritional value to an otherwise entirely nutritionless meal.

I have seen this work well for even the worst of diets. Over time, you will react so positively to these additions that you will begin to crave the healthier items instead of the unhealthy ones. Gradually, those nutritional items that once were merely additions could become the entire focus of your meal.

2. The Replacement Rule

The world is full of tempting treats that create a large amount of craving and satisfaction but offer little nutrition. Traditional favorites such as pizza, ice cream, cookies, sodas, sugared cereal, fast food, and other unhealthy choices are literally addictions and create a real dilemma when trying to make proper decisions. To help avoid caving in to these cravings and addictions, use the Replacement Rule.

Most junk foods contain harmful ingredients such as preservatives, additives, MSG, and hydrogenated oils. However, there are now endless recipes, grain-free and sugar-free alternatives, and products at health food and grocery stores that offer a variety of substitutes you can buy or make that are similar in form, satisfaction, and taste to these foods.

These substitutes are all-natural and at least provide some actual nutrients.

Therefore, to phase out those unhealthy foods that leave you overfed but undernourished, follow the Food Replacement Rule and begin replacing them with more health-conscious substitutes. Replacing fat-, lethargy-, or disease-producing foods with healthful substitutes is an easy and effective way to start to slowly and less painfully change your habits.

Using this rule, you will soon find yourself more and more satisfied with the healthier substitutes to your cravings. Eventually, you may even be able to eliminate these cravings altogether. To help you, here is a handy list of common food cravings and their replacement foods.

Replacement Foods* (See recipes in the back of the book)

Craving/Addiction	Replacement Food
Movie popcorn (Bucket)	Homemade air-popped with olive oil and sea salt
Pizza: Store-bought or homemade	Pizza with almond flour, cauliflower, or zucchini crust recipes, health food store
Ice cream	Make your own! Recipes that use Stevia and even dairy alternatives are abundant and delicious!
Sugary, refined cereal	Grain-free, sugar-free cereal recipe
Sugar	Stevia, Xylitol, unrefined fruit juice, honey, maple syrup

| Rich desserts | Rich desserts using grain-free, sugar-free recipes |

3. THE 10-POINT REDUCTION RULE

If you recall the section about where hunger comes from (Chapter 2: "The Truth About Hunger"), there is a principle called Sensory-Specific Satiety that you can use to your advantage. When you fill up on a certain taste or style of food, your desire for more of it drops considerably.

If on a scale of 1 to 10, if a craving is a 10, it will be hard to resist. On the other hand, if you can get the same craving down to a 7 or 8, you can control cravings some or most of the time. If you can get them down even farther, you can almost totally control them.

Therefore, the 10-Point Reduction Rule states that if you can reduce a food craving to below a level 10, you will have more power over your decisions to consume.

To achieve this elementary rule, it is prudent to start addressing those foods that currently cause a level 10 craving in the first place.

I own this rule personally. I crave something sweet after a meal. Rather than end up with something that will hurt me, we always have cookies, fudge, and brownies from our recipe section handy. This may not be equal to the super-legit cookie loaded with sugar and shortening or Ben & Jerry's, but by eating a healthy recipe or even a piece of fruit I kick my

Sensory-Specific Satiety principle into place, drop the desire to a 7, and can get myself to "just say no."

4. EVERYONE'S FAVORITE: THE VACATION FOOD RULE (OR, THE NEVER DIET AGAIN THEORY)

Rewiring to new habits, as we've covered, takes place over time. So when you say, "I'll never eat bread or have a Margarita again," you may be kidding yourself. It stands to reason that if it took years to build poor eating habits, it will likewise take time to permanently change the wrong eating habits in favor of the right ones.

Studies show that when you say, "I'll never have chocolate again," there is a strong chance for the rebound effect. You'll end up eating twice as much chocolate after your brain goes into survival mode and craves chocolate in order to stay alive.

If eating well creates too much stress, it negates many of the positive benefits, and your new commitments generally go tumbling over a cliff. The Vacation Food Rule was created as a way of making the process of change much less stressful.

In my family growing up, and for the preponderance of the people for whom I've done diet counseling, they were either on a diet program or off it and on a weight-gaining program. Most people are either on a diet or off a diet and believe, "If I cave, I crater." This means that if you eat something off the diet, you're off the diet.

The smartest perspective is The Never Diet Again Theory. You have probably heard someone tell you to make it a lifestyle and not a diet. This is wise. But how do we do that? The Vacation Rule is how. If you have committed to improving your way of eating the rest of your life, then it does not matter if you eat something wrong because the next meal can be right.

Everybody likes a vacation. No matter how satisfying your work is, you need an occasional break. The Vacation Food Rule puts in a food, a meal, or even a whole day of the less-than-ideal food choices as a *rule*. The idea that "if you cave, you crater" is only true for diets. So, rather than calling it "cheating," you intentionally plan a vacation meal or day of eating each week. Or, if you just eat something off the good list because you over-craved one day, then that wasn't cheating either, it was that week's vacation food.

While occasionally you will take a spontaneous vacation, the best vacations are planned. Therefore, suppose you are an ice cream lover. Well, if you eat ice cream every day, not only is that unhealthy, but you are likely going to get fat.

However, if you utilize the Vacation Food Rule, you set a short-term goal for when you *will* eat the ice cream. You may say, "I will eat ice cream only on Wednesdays and Sundays." Then, on Tuesday, when you pass your favorite ice cream parlor or somebody asks if you want to try their cone, you can resist your craving and say, "No thanks, I eat ice cream only on Wednesdays and Sundays."

Some cravings are so great that they are difficult to handle. By setting a short-term goal, you usually can push yourself over the hump and make it another day or two.

It is important to give yourself short vacations from always eating well. However, with the Vacation Food Rule, you may be able to drop some really bad habits entirely. What will eventually happen is that you will be able to put off some of your eating vices longer and longer until eventually you won't desire them at all anymore.

Personally, this rule helped me become addicted to feeling good. And it's done the same for many other people. When I think of many of my old Vacation Rule foods, I anchor more to how lousy I feel after eating them than what they tasted like going down. When you isolate only certain days to eat some of your cravings, you will find that you do not feel well after eating them.

5. THE FOOD DRESS-UP RULE

Initially, many of the healthier food choices may not seem very appealing. God-made foods tend to appear less tasty and fulfilling because of all the additives, sugars, salts, and fats that give less healthy, man-made foods their flavor. The reality is that natural foods do possess good taste, but our taste buds have been dulled due to all the flavorings and spices in man-made food.

In order to make healthy food more palatable to your abused and desensitized taste buds, use the Food Dress-up Rule. With this long-range goal of dressing up meals with healthy alternatives, proper nutrition can be achieved more realistically than by simply eliminating or giving up unhealthy foods altogether.

After a period of using God-made foods, eventually the sensation will return to your taste buds, and foods will require less dressing up. For breakfast, I take the bland, boring, concept of plain yogurt and make it into something I love and eat for breakfast three or four days a week by putting everything in there but the kitchen sink.

Dr. Ben's "Kitchen Sink" Yogurt

Ingredients:

- 1 c. organic whole (or goat's milk) plain yogurt
- 1-2 tsp. shaved unsweetened raw chocolate
- 1/8 tsp. Stevia, to taste
- ¼ c. ground flax seed and/or chia seed pudding
- 1-2 tbsp. shredded coconut (opt.)
- 1 tsp. almond butter
- 1 c. fresh strawberries, raspberries, blueberries, or a combination of mixed berries

6. THE STAY FULL RULE

When we discussed "The Truth About Hunger" in Chapter 2, you may recall that the pangs are not your stomach crying out for nutrients but your body prepping for anticipated digestion along with the brain simply getting psyched to eat. Getting this hungry can really derail your ability to make good choices. That is why the Stay Full Rule states that the way to achieve proper nutrition is not to get too hungry.[8]

I really use this trick as a way of predicting when I'll be hungry so I can avoid getting stuck somewhere without the right kind of food. I always bring food along when traveling, and if I'm going out for a meal or headed to a party, I'll make sure to eat something grain-free and sugar-free first. That way, when I get to my destination I can stick to something small or skip whatever gut-bomb is being served.

Consuming regular, healthy meals at appropriate times of the day achieves a proper balance of staying nourished while also staying satisfied. On the other hand, skipping meals and going hungry leads to a practice of becoming "starved." This creates the need for eating anything within reach to satisfy the inevitable hunger pangs.

What is most satisfying and often most available are those heavily refined fast or fried foods that are full of fat. To avoid consuming such "junk" food, always stay full throughout the day with natural meals and snacks. See the recipe section for great snack ideas (Trick #10: "Recipes For Cheating The System").

TRICK #5: CARB, PROTEIN COUNTER, AND FOOD LISTS

I have written many diet books. This isn't designed to be one of them. But no book on lifestyle would be complete without giving some eating guidance. Having an idea of total carbs and proteins to consume, along with long lists of safe foods, gives you the peace of mind you need to move forward.

Remember the secret: If it's on the safe list, you can load up. But the carbs and sugars aren't on the safe list, so you need to know your limits.

Carb Tricks

Too many carbs will kill any chance you have of reaching weight-loss goals and may even kill you. The trick is knowing your number. In the box below, we show you a range that will work to get you moving in the right direction and provide the carb counter so you can easily do the math.

Diets and Carbohydrate Restriction	
Carbohydrate-restricted (by comparison) diet	125-200 grams per day
Moderately low-carbohydrate diet	75-100 grams per day
Very low-carbohydrate, ketogenic diet (VLCK)	40-50 grams or less per day. As little as 20g in the case of the severely insulin resistant

Here are examples of what these amounts of carbohydrates really look like when you apply them to the real world:

- **VLCK** *(Where many people have to start for weight loss and rebooting hormones. Some stay here long-term.)*: 1 cup of strawberries (11g), ½ cup of almonds (15g), 1 avocado (12g), ½ cup of black beans (12g) = 50g

- **MODERATELY LOW** – A healthy place to start or land long-term depending on carb tolerance: 1 cup of strawberries (11g), sweet potato (24g), ½ cup of peanuts - (12g), ½ cup of chickpeas (27g), and 1 avocado (12g) = 86g

- **CARB RESTRICTED:** Apple (25g), Cup of brown rice (45g), 1 cup of black beans (23g), ½ cup of almonds (15g), and 1 cup of blueberries (21g) = 129 grams

---

CARBOHYDRATES:
EAT IN THE MORNING OR EARLY PART OF THE DAY

One of the fiercest enemies to good health and a lean body is unused carbohydrates. So if you eat a bowl of pasta and some bread at night, you've just eaten enough carbohydrates to run a marathon, but instead you go to bed. These unused carbs wreak havoc on your glands, the abundance of sugars they create overwhelm the insulin mechanisms necessary to absorb them, and they end up stored as fat. All this results in your getting up in the morning feeling more tired than you were when you went to bed. In the morning, it has typically been six to twelve hours since you have fueled up, and you still have an entire day ahead of you. Therefore, energy foods can be used up. So, keeping the majority of your carbs in the morning gives you ample time to burn what you've taken in and leaves little left over for storage in the gut or butt.

THE CARB COUNTER
A Chart of Lower-Glycemic Index Carbohydrate Sources

You don't need to abandon carbohydrates. What follows is a list of low-glycemic carbs and how many grams of carbohydrates they have per serving. It's important to note that in counting carbs, you can subtract total fiber from total carbohydrates. For example, a cup of blackberries has seven net carbs thanks to its 8 grams of fiber.

Food	Serving Size	Total Carbohydrates	Total Fiber
Fruit			
Apples (with skin)	1 medium-sized apple	25	4
Asian Pears	1 whole medium fruit	13	4
Avocado (California)	1 whole, without skin	12	9
Bananas	Medium (7"-8" long)	27	3
Blackberries	1 cup	15	8
Blueberries	1 cup	21	4
Dates (Deglet Nour)	1 cup chopped	110	12
Grapefruit	Full fruit (6"-8" diameter)	26	4
Grapes	1 cup	16	1
Honeydew melon	1 cup balled	16	1
Kiwis	1 cup	26	5
Food	**Serving Size**	**Total Carbohydrates**	**Total Fiber**
Lemons	1 fruit	8	2
Limes	1 lime	7	2
Mangoes	1 cup sliced	28	3

Melon (Cantaloupe)	1 cup balled	16	2
Oranges (Florida)	1 large whole fruit	17	4
Peach	1 large whole	17	3
Pineapple	1 cup, chunked	22	2
Plums	1 fruit	8	1
Pomegranate	1 fruit	53	11
Red cherries	1 cup, without pits	19	2
Strawberries	1 cup whole strawberries	11	3
Tomato	1 large whole	7	2
Watermelon	1 cup balled	12	1
Vegetables			
Artichokes (boiled and prepared)	1 medium artichoke	14	10
Arugula	1 cup, uncooked leaves	1	0
Banana peppers	1 medium whole pepper	2	2
Broccoli	1 cup chopped	6	2
Brussels sprouts	1 cup	8	3
Cabbage	1 cup chopped	5	2
Carrots	1 cup chopped	12	4

Cucumber	1 cup chopped	3	1
Garlic	3 cloves	3	0
Green beans	1 cup	8	4
Green leaf lettuce	1 cup shredded	1	0
Green peas	1 cup	21	7
Jalapeno peppers	1 cup sliced	6	3
Kale	1 cup chopped	7	1
Onions	1 cup chopped	15	3
Potato	1 whole potato	27	2
Pumpkin	1 cup, cubed	8	1
Red peppers	1 medium whole pepper	7	2
Spinach	1 cup, un-cooked leaves	1	1
Summer squash	1 cup sliced	4	1
Sweet corn	1 medium ear	26	3
Sweet potato (cooked, with skin)	1 medium whole	24	4
Swiss chard	1 cup	1	1
Food	**Serving Size**	**Total Carbohydrates**	**Total Fiber**
Artichokes (boiled and prepared)	1 medium artichoke	14	10
Nuts and Legumes			
Almonds	1 cup whole	30	17
Black beans	1 cup	23	8

Brazil nuts	1 cup whole	16	10
Chickpeas (Garbanzo beans)	1 cup	54	11
Lima beans	1 cup	40	9
Macadamia nuts	1 cup whole	19	11
Peanuts	1 cup	24	12
Low-Glycemic, High-Fiber Grains			
Brown rice (cooked)	1 cup	45	4
Multigrain bread	2 slices	22	4
Oats	1 cup	103	17
Quinoa (cooked)	1 cup	39	5
Rye bread	2 slices	30	4

1. Best Low-Carb, Low Glycemic Index (GI) foods: These are the low-carb, low-glycemic winners.

Examples: Asparagus, green pepper, broccoli, Brussels sprouts, cabbage, cauliflower, celery, green beans, lettuces, mushroom, and onion are so high-fiber and low GI (10-15) that they're really "free foods."

2. Good Low-Carb, Low Glycemic Index foods: Eat these foods in morning unless you're young and/or very active.

Examples: Strawberries, blueberries, blackberries, raspberries (Approx. 25)

3. Modest carb, Good Glycemic Index. Eat legumes in moderation. Beans are higher in carbs and GI so best eaten midday with more activity left in the day to burn the carbs and more aggressive rise in sugar. Peanuts are low carb, low Glycemic Index, but still should be eaten only once in a while.

Examples: Legumes: Peanuts (7), Chickpeas (10), and Beans (20-30).

4. Modest carb, Good Glycemic Index: Nuts and seeds

Examples: Sunflower seeds (35), Cashews (27), Almonds (15), Pistachio (15)

5. Starchier foods, mid-moderately high carbs and moderate Glycemic Index. Eat in moderation in the midday. Better a lunch food like beans, with more activity left in the day.

Examples: Carrots (35), Peas (51), Sweet potato (50)

6. Grains, mid-moderate carbs and high Glycemic Index. Best eaten early or when active.

Examples: Brown rice (50), Whole oats (55)

7. Grains, high carb and high Glycemic Index. For the extremely carb tolerant and active.*Examples:* Millet (71), Corn (60), Quinoa (53)

8. Off the charts. Many "healthy" foods have a higher Glycemic Index than many junk foods, and even sugar itself. For Vacation Meals:

- Potato (70-100+)
- White rice (89)
- Instant Oatmeal (83)
- Oven-baked pretzels (83)
- Cream of Wheat (74)
- Bagel (72)
- Whole wheat bread (71)

- Special K, Kellogg's (69)
- vs. Junk Food
- White bread (71)
- Coca-Cola (63)
- Blueberry muffin (60)
- Ice cream, regular (57)
- Snicker's bar (51)
- Peanut M&Ms (33)

GI Source: *health.harvard.edu*

But What About Fruit?

Many fruits have long-enjoyed a reputation as a healthful, wholesome portion of a balanced diet. There are plenty of good reasons for this. After all, fruits come packaged with nutrients, especially vitamins. They're also a good source of dietary fiber, which has no effect on insulin and helps slow the digestion rate of the food so that the sugar isn't introduced to your system all at once.

But that doesn't mean you should load up on fruits; the sugar will catch up to you. The best recommendation is to limit sugar to the morning with a focus on berries first and foremost.

Here's a quick guide to the best and worst fruits when it comes to sugar content:

Low-Sugar Fruits	
Raspberries	Blueberries
Blackberries	Strawberries

High-Sugar Fruits	
Plums	Oranges
Mangos	Bananas
Figs	Pomegranates
Grapes	Cherries

Not only are berries moderate in carbs, they contain many good anti-inflammatory, anti-oxidant, anti-aging phytonutrients.

PROTEIN QUANTITY: HOW MUCH PROTEIN SHOULD YOU EAT?

How much per meal: Conventional science puts the number at which you can absorb protein at a maximum of about 10 grams of protein per hour. Coupled with your liver's limits, you'll be able to synthesize as much as **25-30 grams per meal of protein and no more.** You'll have to wait two to three hours for the effective metabolism of this protein before you can most efficiently take in another dose.

There are different theories out there about the bioavailability of proteins and whether or not your body is forced to digest all of its protein over two to three hours or whether there are longer intestinal transit times.

The bottom line? Once you hit your protein limit, the excess protein isn't helpful or healthy. The body can turn the spillover into blood sugar through a process called "gluconeogenesis." And blood sugar can turn into body fat. That's why you're better off with a smaller amount of protein divided up throughout the day rather than loading up on 50-90 grams in a single sitting.

Choosing Your "Thrive" Protein Levels

As we look to eliminate the carbs, we're left with protein and fat as our sources of energy. A healthy (and higher than standard) amount of protein is an excellent alternative to replacing the sugars, grains, and starches that just turn into sugar anyway. If you're going to get our typical recommendation of protein at 15 percent to 25 percent of your calories, here's what your diet may look like:

Protein Bang For Your Calorie Buck		
Calories	15%-25% of Calories	Grams
1800	270-450	68-113
2000	300-500	75-125
2400	360-600	90-150
2800	420-700	105-180 *

Serious power athletes at 5-6 meals maxed out at 30-35g of protein per meal.

Vegetarians or people without access or the finances to eat well or eat quality protein products should or will lean more to the 15 percent side. Those who are very physically active, such as athletes and bodybuilders, are going to lean more to that 25 percent-plus side.

Within the ranges suggested of 15 percent to 25 percent, there's nothing to support risk of kidney function or the other suggested protein issues like osteoporosis, cancer, dehydration, colon, or liver problems.

To get the right protein levels, just get your 20-30g per meal until you hit your mark.

Example: Protein Choices to Hit Your Mark

4 Eggs (24g) with cheese (6g) = 30g

Protein shake with grass-fed whey and Chia seeds (4g) = 29g

Lunch 5 oz salmon (30g) salad with ground flax seeds (8g) = 38g

Snack of Cashews (5g) and Almonds (7g) = 12g

Dinner – Chicken (32g)

Total protein = 141g

Protein Counter

Here's the information you need to help you determine how to reach 20-30 grams/meal—as well as hit your protein goal throughout the day:

Animal foods	
Land	
Beef average	7g per ounce
4 ounces hamburger	28g
6 ounces steak	42g
3 ounces leg of lamb	22g
3 ounces chicken breast, no skin	24g
4 ounces pork loin	29g
3 ounces cooked ground pork	22g
1 slice bacon	3g
1 slice Canadian bacon	5.5g

Sea	
Fish average	6g per ounce
6 ounce can of Tuna	40g
4 ounces Mahi Mahi	20g

4 ounces Salmon	24-25g
4 ounces Tilapia	23g
3 ounces shrimp	11g
1 ounce Sardines	7g
Eggs and dairy	
Large egg	6g
1 cup milk	8g
½ cup cottage cheese	15g
1 cup yogurt	8-12g (check label)
Soft cheeses (Mozzarella, Brie, etc.)	6g/ounce
Medium cheeses (Cheddar, Swiss)	7.5g/ounce
Hard cheeses (Parmesan)	10g/ounce
Beans, nuts, legumes, and seeds	
2 tablespoons peanut butter	8g
¼ cup Almonds	8g
¼ cup Peanuts	9g
¼ cup Cashews	5g
¼ cup Sunflower seeds	6g
¼ cup Pumpkin seeds	8g
¼ cup Flax seeds	8g
½ cup cooked beans	7-10g average

How to Get 20-30 Grams of Protein in a Meal	
Eggs	4-5 eggs, depending on size
Beef	A 3-4 oz. hamburger patty or beef filet each offers 23-32 grams of protein

Untrimmed steak	3-4 ounces offers 21-28 grams of protein
Leg of lamb	3-4 ounces offers 22-30 grams
Chicken breast, no skin	3-4 ounces offers 24-32 grams
Turkey	3-4 ounces offers 22-30 grams
Mahi Mahi	4-6 ounces offers 20-30 grams
Tilapia	4-6 ounces offers 22.7-31 grams
Salmon	4-6 ounces offers 24-32 grams
Tuna	6 ounce can offers 40 grams of protein
Shrimp	6 ounces offers 22 grams of protein
Milk	Three cups offers 24 grams
Cottage cheese	½ cup offers 15 grams
Soft cheeses (Mozzarella, Brie)	6 grams per ounce
Medium Cheese (Cheddar, Swiss)	7-8 grams per ounce
Hard cheese (Parmesan)	10 grams per ounce

Sources of Good Whole-Food Protein	
Good	Bad
Meat from whole sources like pasture-raised, 100% grass-fed beef, and free-range chicken	Commercial feed- and grain-eating animals injected with growth hormones, steroids, and antibiotics Worse: Processed meats—usually high in Omega 6's and full of nitrites, which can be converted to nitrosamines, a potentially cancer-causing substance Pork and pork products
Wild fish from the "safe fish" list	Farm-raised fish, shell fish, and other fish from the toxic list.
Dairy and eggs from whole, naturally fed sources	Dairy products and eggs from commercial-feed cows and chickens
Seeds: raw flax, hemp, pumpkin, and sunflower seeds	Large amounts of seeds: they're -3 foods, high in Omega 6. Large amounts of roasted seeds.
Moderate amounts of raw walnuts, almonds, cashews	Large amounts! Avoid roasting nuts as well.

Small amounts of fermented soy products	Processed and excessive soy products, i.e., soy milk, soy protein, tofu, etc.
Modest amounts of legumes, including beans, peas, and lentils	Large amounts are a problem due to antinutrients.

Good Proteins for Your Kitchen

1. Safest fish, 2-3 times a week

2. Grass-fed, organic beef

3. Wild game

4. Grass-fed, organic, raw dairy

5. Raw butter and cheese

6. Pasture-raised, free-range chicken and eggs

7. Organic turkey

8. Grass-fed concentrated whey protein (not isolate)

Good Protein for Vegans

- Moderate legumes: beans and lentils

- Raw nuts and seeds

- Vegan plant protein supplement: rice, hemp, pea

- Fermented soy products

If you eat proteins in the right amounts—and from the right sources—you give yourself a great foundation for building muscle and losing fat.

ADD GOOD FATS. LOWER BAD FATS.
Must-have fats in your kitchen:

- Dark, unsweetened chocolate bars
- Unsweetened cocoa powder
- Fish: wild-caught sardines, herring, and salmon
- Fish oil capsules or liquid
- Chia seeds
- Flax seeds
- Avocado
- Almonds
- Pecans
- Pistachios
- Almond butter
- Organic peanut butter
- Extra Virgin Olive Oil
- Extra Virgin Coconut Oil
- Organic, grass-fed butter (Raw is best—at least do organic, as toxins stick to fats)
- Coconut flour
- Almond flour
- Coconut milk
- Whole olives
- Coconut oil
- Organic-, grass-, and finished-fed meats

DON'T BE SCARED

When my youngest son turned four, he learned how to manipulate people (or at least attempt to) by challenging their will. If someone said they didn't want to play with him, or his sister wouldn't share her drink, he'd ask, "Why? Are you scared?"

When you restrict your carbs, you'll be getting more calories from fat. But don't be scared! As we established in previous chapters, it's not dietary fat that makes your butt look fat, clogs your arteries, and packs onto your hips and thighs.

More Eating Fat Tips:

- **Reduce the 6s:** Roasted nuts; vegetable, nut, or seed oils in packaged and prepared foods. Reduce/eliminate commercial meat and dairy products.

- **Add +3s:** Chia or flax seeds in yogurt, smoothies, or on salads, wild-caught salmon or sardines, others from the safe fish list, green vegetables, and an omega supplement.

- **Add monounsaturated (Omega-9) fats:** Extra virgin olive oil on salads instead of commercial dressings, avocados, couple of handfuls of almonds, almond flour, hazelnuts, or macadamia nuts.

- **Medium chain triglycerides:** Coconut milk in your smoothies, cook at moderate heat with coconut oil, recipes using coconut flower.

- **Add saturated fats from good, clean sources:** Although higher in monounsaturated fats than saturated: grass-fed, grass-finished hamburger or steak; pasture-raised and organic chicken and eggs;

organic, grass-fed cheese and butter (raw is best if possible). **Adds Conjugated Linoleic Acid (CLA) which is really good for you as well.**

QUICK CHEAT SHEET

EAT THIS	NOT THIS
Fruit—*Good, Low-Sugar Fruits*: Raspberries, Blackberries, Blueberries, Strawberries *Reduce High-Sugar Fruits*: Plums, Mangos, Figs, Oranges, Bananas, Grapes, Cherries	Concentrated fruit juice, preservative-filled dried fruit
Grains (Eliminate on the Advanced Plan): Ancient grains: Amaranth, Quinoa, Millet, Oatmeal (Gluten-free), Whole-grain rice	Gluten foods: Wheat, Rye, Barley, White Rice, Bread, Pasta
Flour - Coconut Flour, Almond Flour	White, Wheat, Rye, Barley flour
Vegetables, Veggie-Like & Starches: Broccoli, Asparagus, Eggplant, Green beans, Brussels sprouts, Peppers, Onion, Celery, Cucumber, Spinach, Lettuce, Kale, Squash, Zucchini, Snow peas, Mushrooms, Cauliflower, Tomato, Avocado, Sweet Potato (great for recovery)	Corn, Potatoes
Legumes, Seeds, and Nuts: Legumes (Beans, Lentils, Peanuts, and Peas), Raw nuts, Seeds, Nut flour, Chia, *Flax are best,* Sunflower, Pumpkin	Nuts and seeds roasted in vegetable oil. No soy, soy protein, or soy milk. Common GMO foods: soy, canola, sugar beets, corn, wheat, tomatoes, and potatoes.

Sweeteners: Stevia or Xylitol (*in moderation*): Unless you are low carb, can also use raw honey, organic maple syrup, and coconut sugar.	Sucralose (Splenda), Aspartame (NutraSweet), Saccharin, and Maltodextrin
#1 Omega 3s: Chia or flax seeds, safe fish (See list), Green vegetables, Omega supplement	Vegetable, Nut, and Seed oils, Commercial meat and dairy, Oils in packaged foods
Monounsaturated (Omega-9) fats: Extra virgin olive oil, avocados, almonds, almond flour, hazelnuts or macadamia nuts. **Good Fat = Lose Fat & Inflammation**	Trans-fats **Bad Fat = Get Fat & Inflamed**
Olive oil-based dressings	Vegetable- or canola-based, high-sugar and high-calorie dressings
Coconut milk, coconut oil, coconut flower	
Good saturated fats from properly raised sources: Grass-fed beef (hamburger or steak); pasture-raised and organic chicken and eggs; organic, grass-fed cheese and butter (raw is best if possible)	Limit fats from commercial meats and commercial dairy products.
The best oils for cooking Coconut oil, butter oil. Olive oil (low temperature or cold only)	**Bad for cooking or use at any time** Vegetable, nut, or seed oil
Dairy Organic, grass-fed dairy products; goat's milk dairy products; organic, raw butter and cheese; grass-fed, undenatured whey powder	Any non-organic commercial dairy product. No commercial cheese, milk, whey

Beverages: Purified water (can add lemon), lemon and Stevia, cucumber slices, sparkling water (with lemon or lime), fresh vegetable juices, smoothies (see recipes)	*No* **Soda: Diet or Regular** No commercial dairy Limit caffeine and alcohol Apple, orange, grape, grapefruit juice, etc.
Meat from whole sources like pasture-raised, 100% grass-fed and finished beef, and free-range chicken	Commercial feed and grain-eating animals injected with growth hormones, steroids, and antibiotics *Worse*: Processed meats Pork and pork products
Wild fish from the "safe fish" list	Farm-raised fish, shell fish, and other fish from the toxic list
Dairy and eggs from whole, naturally fed sources	Dairy products and eggs from commercial, feed cows, and chickens
Seeds: raw flax, hemp, pumpkin, and sunflower seeds	Large amounts of seeds Large amounts of roasted seeds
Moderate amounts of raw walnuts, almonds, cashews	Large amounts! Avoid roasting nuts as well.
Small amounts of fermented soy products	Processed and excessive soy products, i.e., soy milk, soy protein, tofu, etc.
Modest amounts of legumes: including beans, peas, and lentils.	Large amounts are a problem due to anti-nutrients.

Good Protein for Vegans:	Do not eat or drink soy!
Moderate legumes: beans and lentils	
Raw nuts and seeds	
Vegan plant protein supplement: rice, hemp, peas	
Fermented soy product	

TRICK #6: SNACK IT UP, DESSERT IT UP!
Snacks

One way to really crave carbs is to get to the point where you're starving and ready to eat a hippo. The key with snacks is to avoid starvation while not adding carbs between meals. If you have an after-dinner snack, it should be eaten two to three hours before bed—although vegetables are always "free" even right before bedtime. If you're perfectly satisfied or struggling to lose weight, then you don't need to eat between meals or after dinner.

Snack Suggestions

- Granny Smith apple alone or with 1-2 tbsp almond or peanut butter. Nut butters should have no added ingredients—just the nut.

- Celery with 1-2 tbsp of almond or peanut butter or organic cream cheese

- Vegetable sticks (celery, cucumber, green/red/yellow pepper, Romaine) with hummus, yogurt veggie dip,* guacamole, or hummus

- ½ cup of Greek or goat's milk yogurt with Stevia to taste, shredded coconut, shaved unsweetened chocolate, and ground flax seeds or chia seeds

- Green smoothie

- The dessert recipes—remember, they're made of nut flowers, good fats, and nonsugar sweeteners, so they're a food.

- Mixed sweet nuts*

- Raw almonds, pistachios, peanuts (on occasion), hazelnuts, and pecans. Cashews are higher on the Glycemic Index (So not great for low carb)

- Salads and leftover cooked proteins and vegetables

- Chocolate Malted Smoothie*

- Breakfast recipes such as Grainless Granola* and Brownie Cereal* and dessert recipes such as Chocolate Avocado Pudding or Chocolate Chia Pudding* or no-guilt Gooey Chocolate Chip Cookies* make for great snacks!

- (*See Recipes section in Trick #10.)

Desserts

Desserts in our plan provide limited carbs and can be eaten for snacks and after meals. We've placed something sweet after dinner in the plan, but it's not an absolute. Again, if satisfied, it's your choice to partake or not.

Supplement Guide & Guidance

High quality, whole-food supplements should make up a part of your regular nutrition plan. You just don't get the nutrients you need for optimum functioning from diet alone. Twenty-five years of practice and analyzing hundreds of thousands of patients has led me and the other doctors I work with to recommend a certain supplement baseline. These include:

- A daily detoxification supplement
- Vitamin D
- An omega fatty acid supplement
- Women's or men's multivitamin
- A daily anti-inflammatory supplement
- A greens product
- Grass-fed whey or the vegetarian alternative

Some Explanation of the Maximizing Cooking and Meal Plans

One way to cut costs, make it easier, and increase convenience is to cook enough of one meal for two or three meals at a time. Then, the next day, you eat the leftovers—which are almost always better the second day—rather than having to cook again.

Leftovers also make great snacks. If you're hungry between meals or after dinner, you can eat leftovers—which you know are safe and fit the plan.

On a tight budget? Look for the Cost Conscious meals in the recipe section that follows the Food List in Trick #9.

The following meal plans ensure that if you, someone in your family, or someone who cooks for you likes to shop and prepare recipes, then you can create great-tasting dishes with tons of variety. Or, you may simply like the basics for "staple" meals.

Staple Meal Example—My Staple Foods

- Breakfast: eggs, smoothies, or unsweetened yogurt sweetened with Stevia, berries, and other healthy additions.

- Lunch: Salads with protein, olive oil dressings, and healthy, raw and/or organic cheeses.

- Snacks: Granny Smith apples, raw nuts and seeds, and grain-free/sugar-free desserts.

- Dinner: Chicken/fish/grass-fed meat, salad, and steamed or stir-fried vegetables, grain-free, sugar-free dessert

We've named specific meals, snacks, and dessert examples in the plan (coming up in Trick #10), but you can choose from the many recipes we've provided that are listed by breakfast, lunch, dinner, or snack. It's all about mixing, matching, and making this plan work for you!

TRICK #7: LEARN HOW TO READ A LABEL
How to Read a Food Label

Law dictates that each food label gives you the same information in the same place every single time. That's the good news; it keeps things simple. The bad news is not all of the information is very relevant, which means you'll have to do a little learning on your own in order to understand which numbers on the food label really matter.

```
Nutrition Facts
Serving Size ¾ cup (55g)
Servings Per Container 5
```

Amount Per Serving	
Calories 250	Calories from Fat 50

	% Daily Value*
Total Fat 6g	**9%**
Saturated Fat 0.5g	**3%**
Cholesterol <5mg	**<2%**
Sodium 200mg	**8%**
Total Carbohydrate 40g	**13%**
Dietary Fiber 4g	**16%**
Sugars 18g	
Protein 9g	**18%**

Vitamin A 25% • Vitamin C 50% • Calcium 30% • Iron 25%
*Percent Daily Values based on a 2,000 Calorie diet.

- **% Daily Value.** A child, an adult with diabetes, an endurance athlete, someone who sits at a desk all day, a pregnant mother, and a grandfather all have *substantially* different nutrient needs. Therefore, the "Daily Values" expressed on food labels are of very little informative value to you. When reading as "% Daily Value" or "%DV," you should ask, "Daily Value for *whom*?"

- **Total Carbs, Fats, and Proteins.** This is good, relevant information, and it's what you need to start checking on all of your food. After listing total Calories, the next bolded items include Total Fat, Cholesterol, Sodium, Total Carbohydrate, and Proteins. For the purpose of following the plans, figure out the percentage. Remember, carbs and proteins contain 4 calories/gram and fat contains 9 calories per gram. In the included food label example, there are 250 calories made up of:

> Carbs: 31g x 4cal/g = 124 calories
> Protein: 5g x 4cal/g = 20 calories
> Fats: 2g x 9 cal/g = 108 calories
> **So carbs make up 50% of this food.**

- **Ingredients list.** Food manufacturers have to list their ingredients, which means you'll know exactly what you're putting in your body. A good rule of thumb? The *fewer* ingredients listed here, the better; and if you don't understand the words, don't eat the ingredients.

- **Serving size.** This is another variable to watch out for. You might think a food has few trans-fats, carbs, or calories, only to see that the serving size is the equivalent of a thimble-full. Looking at the serving size first, at the top of the food label, is a great way to understand the overall "context" for all of the numbers printed below.

Manufacturers like to draw your attention away from the nutrition facts by advertising a "healthful" ingredient on the front of the box. They'll tell you all about their product's "whole-grain goodness" or "heart-healthy ingredients." But what they don't advertise are the *other* ingredients present: processed grains, chemicals, colorings, and enough sweeteners to flavor your swimming pool. Once you read the ingredients list, you have to make a choice: Too many sugars? Too many carbs? Chemical ingredients? If the answer is yes, then just say, "No." Even if the package claims it's healthy.

TRICK #8: EXECUTIVE STRATEGIES FOR SUCCESS
Goals

What goals, aspirations, desires, and intentions do you want to accomplish in the first 30 days of lifestyle change?

Diet

_____

_____

_____

Exercise

_____

_____

_____

Health

_____

_____

_____

Social

_____

_____

_____

Sleep

_____

_____

_____

Work

_____

_____

_____

DON'T MAKE FANTASY GOALS

The ideal is that we lock on to the end result and never, ever quit. On the other hand, you may have quit before. If so:

- What would motivate you to start again?
- What would cause you to stop doing it, even if it did?
- What would make you start doing it again, even if you stopped for that reason?
- What would cause you to stop again?

These are some probing questions to ask yourself. Hopefully the answers you give to the motivators and stops will push you to prepare to keep pushing through.

Begin Your Three-Day Diet Diary

Because food makes such an impact on the quality and quantity of your life, it is essential to know what you are already eating. Believe it or not, most people do not realize what they are putting in their mouths each day. Only by recording everything you eat over a period of time can you truly evaluate the kinds of foods you are eating, the amount of food you are eating, and the moods you are experiencing before and after eating. In order for you to get a good picture of exactly where you stand, we will begin a Three-Day Diet Diary.

THREE-DAY DIET DIARY
Day 1

1. Record the time of all food, beverage, vitamin, or medication intake.

2. Record the approximate size and amount of each item.

3. Record WHY you are eating. (Bored, Tired, Hungry, Social, Business, Time, Depressed, etc.)

4. Record how you FELT after eating. How did you feel one hour after eating?

5. Please note if there is a time of day when you are particularly stressed, tired, or in a lot of pain.

Day 2

1. Record the time of all food, beverage, vitamin, or medication intake.

2. Record the approximate size and amount of each item.

3. Record WHY you are eating. (Bored, Tired, Hungry, Social, Business, Time, Depressed, etc.)

4. Record how you FELT after eating. How did you feel one hour after eating?

5. Please note if there is a time of day when you are particularly stressed, tired, or in a lot of pain.

Day 3

1. Record the time of all food, beverage, vitamin, or medication intake.

2. Record the approximate size and amount of each item.

3. Record WHY you are eating. (Bored, Tired, Hungry, Social, Business, Time, Depressed, etc.)

4. Record how you FELT after eating. How did you feel one hour after eating?

5. Please note if there is a time of day when you are particularly stressed, tired, or in a lot of pain.

Now write down your favorite foods that you could see putting in your diet every week. List them by category—fats, carbohydrates, or proteins:

_____

_____

_____

_____

PUTTING THE PLAN TOGETHER CREATING SOLID YELLOW BOXES

Busy, successful people can stay focused. They compartmentalize their time so they can get multiple things done better than many people can get *one* thing done. They are able to focus. Focus in a war means you can't be looking at or thinking about something else. Your total energies are centered on the battle at hand. Being distracted can be the difference between success and failure, life or death. When you're putting time into an area of your life, it also needs focused energy.

What you need to do as you formulate your personal War Plan is draw lines around each one of your lives. Think of it like this: When you are driving, if you see a dotted yellow line, it means you can pass or cross over into the other lane. Here, you put solid yellow lines around any area of health for which you have a goal.

If you paint solid yellow lines around each of your lives and the To-Do's they contain, other lives cannot pass or cross over.

SOLID YELLOW LINE EXAMPLES
Monday

7 a.m.–7:10 a.m. FITNESS LIFE—SURGE TRAINING

From 7 a.m.–7:10 a.m. you put yourself in the yellow box of Surge Training.

9 a.m.–1 p.m. Financial Life

Put yourself in the yellow box of your chosen occupation. By focusing on your work and not your eight other lives, along with a dozen other distractions, you'll succeed and more than likely vastly improve your financial prospects. No other life is allowed in at that time. No personal calls, no exercise "breaks," no personal growth at that time. Do not look at an e-mail.

1:15 p.m.–2:30 p.m. DATE LUNCH WITH SPOUSE

Here you put yourself in the yellow box of Family Life. Fully concentrate on your spouse during this time. Don't let colleagues intrude on your time. Don't answer your cell phone. Stay in your yellow box.

2:45 p.m.–5:45 p.m. FINANCIAL LIFE

6:30 p.m.–9:15 p.m. FAMILY LIFE

From 6 o'clock until 9:15 each evening, there's a very impenetrable solid-yellow family box. Again, you're in the box. This means relational time—no TV, no cell phones, no Internet. That's quality, present time. Plus, by making sure this time is penciled firmly in place, consistently each day, it becomes quantity, present time. If you want strong relationships and healthy children who don't grow up to quit college and take drugs, then you need quality and quantity focused time.

9:15 p.m.–10 p.m. EDUCATION AND PERSONAL-GROWTH LIFE

Study a book or computer program designed to advance learning in an area important to the advancement of your personal life. This could also be time for relaxation or going to sleep.

Not every minute has something in it, but ideally every "life" you live is scheduled. Sometimes it's nap life, but it's still scheduled. (I learned that one in kindergarten.) Certain lives you live happen every day, but others are strategically placed throughout the week. This is so all the items on your written To-Do list are checked off and done *well*.

Obviously, it doesn't always work out so perfectly. Sometimes a child wakes up during times designated for something else besides changing a diaper or an extremely urgent issue pops up that cannot be handled by the people who now help you in life. At those times, you have to practice flexibility. If other people's lives cross over your double yellow lines into one of your lives, as they occasionally will, try to remember the admonition, "That's life." Work to get past the issues and try to get everyone and everything back in their lanes as quickly as possible before there is an accident!

Unfortunately, a few times a year there are some traumatic, stressful Five Lives pileups. But by getting back to healthy compartmentalization through the building of solid yellow boxes and proper delegation, you can usually manage to escape with only some minor damage.

TRICK #9: THE FOOD LIST–PULL FROM THIS AND YOU'LL DO WELL
Food Lists

This contains some of the common foods and ingredients eaten for breakfast, lunch, dinner, and snacks.

Breakfast

Low-carb foods:

- Almond, coconut flour
- Avocado
- Blackberries
- Blueberries
- Cheese

- Cheeses (*organic recommended*)
- Chia seed
- Coconut milk
- Eggs
- Flax seed
- Goat's milk or organic yogurt
- Granny Smith apples
- Grass-fed dairy products
- Organic butter
- Raspberries
- Raw nuts*, seeds*, nut butter (*without added oils or sugars*)
- Smoothies
- Stevia
- Strawberries
- Vegan protein powder: hemp, pea, brown rice
- Vegetables
- Whey powder

Best carbs to eat when eating carbs:

- Ancient grains*: Amaranth, Quinoa, and Millet
- Higher sugar fruits: Bananas, grapes, pineapple, red apples, plums, watermelon
- Oatmeal (gluten-free)
- Raw, organic honey, coconut sugar, organic maple syrup

Lunch

Low-carb foods:

- Almond, coconut flour
- Avocado
- Berries
- Carrots
- Cheeses (*organic recommended*)
- Chia seeds
- Extra virgin coconut oil
- Extra virgin olive oil
- Flax seeds
- Granny Smith apples
- Grapeseed-oil dressing
- Green smoothies
- Legumes* (beans, lentils, peanuts, peas, etc.)
- Nut butter (*without added oils or sugars*)
- Raw nuts*, seeds*, and nut flour.
- Safe fish (*see list*)
- Salads
- Steak/beef/chicken (*organic recommended*)
- Vegetables

Best carbs to eat when eating carbs:

- Ancient grains*: amaranth, quinoa, and millet
- Brown rice

- Higher sugar fruits: bananas, grapes, pineapple, red apples, plums, watermelon
- Sweet potato

Dinner

Low-carb foods:

- Almond, coconut flour
- Asparagus
- Avocado
- Broccoli
- Brussels sprouts
- Cabbage
- Cauliflower
- Cheeses (*organic recommended*)
- Extra virgin coconut oil
- Extra virgin olive oil
- Safe fish: sardines, tilapia, salmon, flounder, herring
- Salads
- Steak/chicken (*organic recommended*)
- Vegetables

Best carbs to eat when eating carbs (Limit or eliminate at dinner—you're going to sleep and don't need carbs!):

- Ancient grains*: amaranth, quinoa, and millet
- Brown rice
- Legumes* (beans, lentils, peanuts, peas, etc.)
- Fruit

TRICK #10: RECIPES FOR CHEATING THE SYSTEM

I eat so many desserts, my kids tell me I'm cheating the system. However, it's not just a dietetic meal or dessert—the recipes that follow contain nutrients that are good for you.

chapter 7

BREAKFAST AND SMOOTHIE RECIPES

BERRY BREAKFAST SMOOTHIE

Servings: 1 (Serving Size: 1 (8 oz.) green smoothie)
Total Time – Prep to Finish: 5 minutes

Ingredients

- 1 c. fresh berries of choice (strawberries, blackberries, raspberries, etc., or a combination of mixed berries)
- ½ c. coconut milk
- ½ c. crushed ice and/or water (as needed for desired thickness)
- 1 scoop Vanilla Perfect Protein powder
- ½ c. flax seeds and/or chia seeds

Directions

- In a blender, combine the contents and process until smooth, adding more crushed ice or water as needed to achieve desired thickness.

- Pour the smoothie into a tall glass and drink immediately to receive full nutritional value – the nutrients will begin to dissipate the longer the smoothie is exposed to the air.

Nutritional Data

Calories: 278

Total Fat: 20 (saturated: 10; polyunsaturated: 4.3; monounsaturated: 1.1)

Carbohydrates: 17

Fiber: 7

Protein: 8

●●●

CHOCOLATE-COVERED STRAWBERRY SMOOTHIE

Servings: 1 (Serving Size: 1 (8 oz.) green smoothie)
Total Time – Prep to Finish: 5 minutes

Ingredients

- ½ c. coconut milk

- 1-2 c. crushed ice, depending on desired thickness/consistency

- ½ avocado, peeled, stone removed and discarded; flesh chopped

- 1½ c. fresh strawberries, hulled and quartered
- 2-3 tbsp. unsweetened cocoa powder
- 1 scoop Chocolate Perfect Protein powder

Directions

1. In a blender, combine the contents and process until smooth, adding more crushed ice or water as needed to achieve desired thickness.

2. Pour the smoothie into a tall glass and drink immediately to receive full nutritional value – the nutrients will begin to dissipate the longer the smoothie is exposed to the air.

Nutritional Data

Calories: 489
Total Fat: 41
Carbohydrates: 37
Fiber: 16
Protein: 9

•••

NUTRITION KNOCK-OUT GREEN SMOOTHIE

Servings: 1 (Serving Size: 1 (8 oz.) green smoothie)
Total Time – Prep to Finish: 5 minutes

Ingredients

- 1 c. filtered water

- 1 c. fresh strawberries, hulled and quartered
- 2 c. romaine lettuce, chopped
- 2 tbsp. lemongrass, chopped
- ½ tsp. ground flaxseed
- 1 scoop Vanilla Perfect Protein powder
- 4-6 ice cubes, or as needed

Directions

1. In a blender, combine the coconut water, strawberries, romaine lettuce, lemongrass, and the ice cubes.

2. Process just until smooth and then add in the ground flaxseed and protein powder; process again for 5-10 seconds or until well incorporated.

3. Add additional ice, if needed until desired consistency is achieved.

4. Pour the green smoothie into tall glass and drink immediately to receive full nutritional value – the nutrients will begin to dissipate the longer the smoothie is exposed to the air.

Nutritional Data

Calories: 77
Total Fat: 1.1
Carbohydrates 17
Fiber: 4
Protein: 9

•••

CHERRY VANILLA GREEN SMOOTHIE

Servings: 1 (Serving Size: 1 (8 oz.) smoothie)
Total Time – Prep to Finish: 5 minutes

Ingredients

- ½ c. coconut milk
- 1-2 c. organic frozen cherries, pitted
- 1 c. spirulina (opt)
- 1 c. raw spinach
- 1 scoop Vanilla Perfect Protein Powder
- ½ c. So Delicious (or preferred brand) dairy-free coconut milk-based Greek yogurt, vanilla flavored
- 5-6 ice cubes (opt.)

Directions

1. Place the coconut milk, cherries, spirulina, yogurt, and the ice (opt.) into the blender. Cover and blend until smooth, stopping frequently to push down any ingredients that may have stuck to the blender walls.

2. Pour into a tall glass and drink immediately to receive full nutritional value.

Nutritional Data

Calories: 354
Total Fat: 29
Carbohydrates: 24
Fiber: 6
Protein: 5

•••

STRAWBERRIES AND SPINACH GREEN SMOOTHIE

Cost Conscious Meal: A pint of strawberries and one bunch of baby spinach costs less than $5 dollars and can be divided and spread out to make smoothies, such as this one; as well as simple salads, sandwiches/wraps, and many more meals.

Servings: 1 (Serving Size: 1 (8 oz.) smoothie)
Total Time – Prep to Finish: 5 minutes

Ingredients

- 1 c. baby spinach
- 2 c. fresh strawberries, hulled and quartered
- 1 scoop Vanilla Perfect Protein Powder
- ½ avocado, peeled
- ½-1 c. coconut water (or filtered water)
- 1 c. crushed ice, as needed to achieve desired thickness

Directions

1. Place ingredients in blender in order listed.

2. Cover and blend until smooth, stopping frequently to push down any ingredients that may have stuck to the blender walls.

3. Pour into a tall glass and drink immediately to receive full nutritional value.

Nutritional Data

Calories: 304

Total Fat: 30

Carbohydrates: 31

Fiber: 13

Protein: 5

•••

SPINACH AND EGG OMELET

Servings: 2 (Serving Size: 1 omelet)
Total Time – Prep to Finish: 20 minutes

Ingredients

- 2 large pasture-raised eggs
- 1 c. baby spinach, chopped or torn
- Sea salt, to taste
- Fresh ground black pepper, to taste
- 1 tsp. coconut oil

Directions

- Place a 10-inch non-stick skillet over medium-low heat. Melt the coconut oil in the skillet.

- In a small bowl, whisk together the eggs, salt, and black pepper. Pour the beaten egg into the skillet, and swirl the pan around to help spread the egg out.

- When the egg is nearly set, but still has a little raw egg left on the surface, sprinkle on the torn spinach and then use a spatula to carefully peel up the edges of the eggs and fold the egg in half. Continue cooking until egg is set. Then transfer to plate and enjoy!

Nutritional Data

Calories: 207
Total Fat: 13
Carbohydrates: 2
Fiber: 0
Protein: 12

•••

2 EGGS AND AN AVOCADO

Cost Conscious Meal: A dozen eggs can make for easy, cost-effective meals that can be very versatile.

Servings: 1 (Serving Size: (2 eggs; 1 avocado)
Total Time – Prep to Finish: 10 minutes

Ingredients

- 2 large pasture-raised eggs, cooked to order

- 1/2-1 ripe avocado, sliced

Directions

1. In a 10-inch nonstick skillet or frying pan, cook eggs according to preference.

2. Slice the avocado and serve alongside the eggs.

Nutritional Data

Calories: 205
Total Fat: 19
Carbohydrates: 9
Fiber: 7
Protein: 2

●●●

SCRAMBLED EGGS WITH APPLE

Servings: 1 (Serving Size: 2 eggs, ½ apple)
Total Time – Prep to Finish: 10 minutes

Ingredients

- 2 large pasture-raised eggs

- ½ Granny Smith apple, cored and cut into wedges

- sea salt, or to taste

- fresh ground black pepper, or to taste

Directions

1. Do not cut the apple until ready to serve to keep the wedges fresh.

2. Place the eggs into a shallow bowl with the salt and black pepper. Whisk lightly just until beaten, then pour the beaten egg into the empty side of the skillet and scramble for about 3-5 minutes or until desired doneness is achieved.

3. Now, it is time to core and wedge the apple, and then arrange ½ of the apple wedges alongside the eggs. Sprinkle with additional sea salt and black pepper, if needed to taste, and then serve and enjoy.

Nutritional Data

Calories: 168
Total Fat: 8
Carbohydrates: 14
Fiber: 2
Protein: 12

●●●

FRIED EGGS AND CHERRY TOMATOES

Servings: 1 (Serving Size: 2 eggs; 1 c. cherry tomatoes)
Total Time – Prep to Finish: 10 minutes

Ingredients

- ½ tbsp. coconut oil
- sea salt, to taste

- fresh ground black pepper, to taste
- 2 large pasture-raised eggs
- 1 c. cherry tomatoes

Directions

1. Heat the ½ tbsp. coconut oil in a skillet, and let melt over medium heat. Add the eggs and space them about 1 inch apart. Sprinkle lightly, to season, with sea salt and black pepper. Cook until desired doneness is achieved.

2. Place the fried eggs on a serving plate, and serve alongside 1 c. cherry tomatoes.

Nutritional Data

Calories: 205
Total Fat: 15
Carbohydrates: 8
Fiber: 2
Protein: 13

●●●

"KITCHEN SINK" YOGURT

Cost Conscious Meal: A simple, inexpensive breakfast of yogurt and fresh berries costs less than $2.00 per serving!

*Servings: 1 (Serving Size: (1 c. yogurt; 1 c. fresh berries)
Total Time – Prep to Finish: 5 minutes*

Ingredients

- 1 c. organic whole (or goat's milk) plain yogurt
- 1-2 tsp. shaved unsweetened raw chocolate
- 1/8 tsp. Stevia, to taste
- ¼ c. ground flax seed and/or chia seeds
- 1-2 tbsp. shredded coconut (opt.)
- 1 tsp. almond or peanut butter
- 1 c. fresh strawberries, raspberries, blueberries, or a combination of mixed berries

Directions

1. Combine all ingredients except for the fresh berries into a bowl. Stir to mix well
2. Fold in ½ of the berries, and stir gently. Then sprinkle the top of the yogurt with the remaining berries.
3. Enjoy!

Nutritional Data

Calories: 325
Total Fat: 17
Carbohydrates: 32
Fiber: 11
Protein: 11

●●●

VEGETABLE AND EGG BREAKFAST SCRAMBLE

Servings: 1 (Serving Size: 2 scrambled eggs with veggies)
Total Time – Prep to Finish: 15 minutes

Ingredients

- 2 large pasture-raised eggs
- ¼ c. white onion, chopped
- ½ c. raw spinach, chopped fine (opt.)
- sea salt, or to taste
- white pepper, or to taste

Directions

1. In a small mixing bowl, add the eggs and beat lightly; whisk in the sea salt and white pepper.

2. Place a medium-sized nonstick skillet over medium-low heat. Pour the beaten eggs into the skillet and cook, stirring often, for 3-5 minutes or until the eggs begin to scramble. When the eggs are nearly done, toss in the veggies, and gently stir to incorporate. Continue cooking until eggs are set, vegetables are heated through, and the spinach is slightly wilted.

3. Transfer the scrambled eggs to a serving dish, sprinkle on a little more sea salt and white pepper, if desired, to taste, and then serve immediately.

Nutritional Data

Calories: 136
Total Fat: 8
Carbohydrates: 5
Fiber: 1
Protein: 13

●●●

2 EGGS AND FRESH BERRIES

Servings: 1 (Serving Size: 2 eggs; 1 c. fresh berries)
Total Time – Prep to Finish: 10 minutes

Ingredients

- 2 large pasture-raised eggs, cooked as desired
- 1 c. fresh berries

Directions

1. In a 10-inch nonstick skillet or frying pan, cook eggs according to preference.
2. Rinse 1 c. of fresh berries and serve alongside the eggs.

Nutritional Data

Calories: 200
Total Fat: 9
Carbohydrates: 19
Fiber: 5
Protein: 13

•••

EGGNOG SMOOTHIE (1 SERVING)

Ingredients

- 2 Whey protein powder (approximately 15 g protein)
- ½ Can coconut milk (full-fat)
- ½ Avocado
- 1-2 Cups ice (for desired thickness and consistency)
- 2 Capfuls vanilla extract
- 2 Tsp ground nutmeg and cinnamon
- Stevia to taste

Directions

Add all ingredients into the blender. Blend on high until creamy and frothy. Serve immediately.

•••

GRAINLESS GRANOLA (2 SERVINGS)

Ingredients

- ¼ cup whole organic flax seeds
- ¼ cup raw organic almonds
- ¼ cup dry, unsweetened coconut
- 2 tsp dried mint leaves or 2 mint tea bags
- ½ cup chilled coconut milk

Directions

1. In blender or food processor, pour flax seeds, almonds, and dry coconut through opening in top of cover. Replace removable cap, and continue processing until ingredients are reduced to a chunky, grain-like consistency, about 1 minute. Stop motor, and scrape down to loosen mixture in bottom of blender or bowl, if necessary.

2. Add loose, dry mint leaves, or open 2 mint tea bags, and dump contents. Process a few more bursts until blended.

3. Can be enjoyed cold, or let stand a few minutes, and warm slightly on stovetop for a "hot" cereal experience. Flax seeds will thicken mixture as it sits.

Nutritional Data

Calories: 265
Fat: 20 grams (6 grams monounsaturated, 10 grams saturated, 5 grams polyunsaturated)
Carbohydrates: 12 grams
Fiber: 8 grams
Protein: 9 grams

●●●

BLUEBERRY MUFFINS (10 MUFFINS)
Ingredients

- 3 organic eggs
- ½ cup whole milk Greek yogurt
- 1/3 cup grapeseed oil

- ½ cup Xylitol
- 1 Tbsp. vanilla extract
- ½ cup coconut flour
- ¼ tsp sea salt
- ¼ tsp baking soda
- 1 cup fresh or frozen blueberries

Directions

1. Preheat oven to 350, and line muffin tins.
2. In a food processor combine eggs, yogurt, oil, vanilla and Xylitol. Pulse until mixed.
3. Pulse in coconut flour, salt, and baking soda. Add blueberries, and pulse two or three times to break up slightly.
4. Fill lined muffin tins. Bake for 20-25 minutes until tops are slightly browned. Makes 10 muffins.

Nutritional data (per muffin)

Calories: 145
Fat: 10 (5 grams monounsaturated, 3 grams saturated, 2 grams polyunsaturated)
Carbohydrates: 9
Fiber: 4
Protein: 5

●●●

BROWNIE CEREAL

Ingredients

- 1 1/2 cups unsweetened shredded coconut
- 1/3 cup unsweetened coconut milk
- 1/4 cup unsweetened cocoa powder
- 1/2 teaspoon liquid or powder Stevia to taste
- 1/2 teaspoon vanilla extract

Directions

1. Preheat oven to 350F.
2. Blend the coconut milk and coconut powder in a stainless steel pot at medium heat.
3. Add in the Stevia and shredded coconut until it's all blended in, and remove from heat.
4. Spread mixture into a thin layer on a parchment on a baking sheet.
5. Bake at 350F for 25-30 minutes dependent on how crunchy you like it.
6. Stir the granola about 15 minutes, and make sure it doesn't burn. Store in airtight container.

●●●

COCONUT PANCAKES WITH BLUEBERRIES

Servings: 1 (Serving Size: 2 pancakes)
Total Time – Prep to Finish: 10 minutes

Ingredients

- 1 pasture-raised eggs
- ¼ c. coconut milk
- ¼ c. water
- ½ tsp baking soda
- ¼ c. coconut flour
- ¼ c. fresh blueberries
- 1 tbsp. unsweetened shredded coconut (opt.)
- ½ tbsp. coconut oil

Directions

1. In a large mixing bowl, combine the eggs, coconut milk, water, baking soda, and coconut flour. Whisk contents together just until blended and a good pancake batter is formed – be careful to not over mix.

2. Fold in the blueberries and coconut (if using) until incorporated. Let batter sit for a couple minutes while you prepare the griddle.

3. Heat a griddle with coconut oil over medium heat. When the oil has melted, pour ¼ c. batter onto the griddle. Fit as many pancakes on the griddle as possible without them touching and still allowing enough room to be able to flip each pancake with a spatula.

4. Let the pancakes cook for 3-4 minutes, then when bubbles appear along the surface, flip the pancakes and cook the other side for 2-3 minutes or until golden brown.

5. Serve and enjoy.

Nutritional Data

Calories: 364
Total Fat: 27
Carbs: 14
Dietary Fiber: 2
Sugars: 8
Protein: 7

●●●

WAFFLES WITH MIXED BERRIES

Servings: 1 (Serving Size: 2 waffles)
Total Time – Prep to Finish: 10 minutes

Ingredients

- ¼ c. blanched almond flour
- 1/8 c. tapioca starch (or arrowroot powder, if preferred)
- 1/8 tbsp. + 1/8 tsp. baking powder
- ½ tbsp. coconut palm sugar
- 1/8 tsp. sea salt, or to taste
- 1 pasture-raised egg
- ½ tbsp. coconut oil, melted
- 1/8 c. coconut milk
- ¼ tsp. fresh-squeezed lemon juice
- ¼ tsp. vanilla extract

- ½ tbsp. almond butter (or preferred toppings)
- ¼ c. fresh mixed berries of choice (blueberries, strawberries, raspberries, blackberries, etc.)

Directions

1. Preheat your waffle iron.

2. In a mixing bowl, combine all of the ingredients in the order listed (except for the almond butter and mixed berries) and mix until just barely combined, a few remaining lumps are fine. Let the waffle batter sit at room temperature for 5 minutes.

3. Using a ladle, scoop approximately ¼ c. of the batter (or the amount indicated by the waffle iron's manufacturer) onto your hot waffle iron. Cook the waffles according to the manufacturer directions for your particular waffle iron or for 4-6 minutes or until your preferred doneness/crispiness is reached.

4. Place the 2 waffles on a serving plate, add on the almond butter or desired toppings and then top the waffles with the fresh mixed berries. Note: For super-quick breakfasts, make a large batch of waffles and freeze them. Then, just pull them out of the freezer and place in the toaster or toaster oven to reheat.

Nutritional Data

Calories: 225
Total Fat: 16
Carbs: 21
Dietary Fiber: 2
Sugars: 8
Protein: 10

chapter 8

LUNCH RECIPES

GRILLED CHICKEN CHOPPED SALAD

Servings: 1 (Serving Size: 2 c. salad with 4-6 grilled chicken)
Total Time – Prep to Finish: 20 minutes

Ingredients

- 4-6 oz. free-range boneless, skinless chicken breast
- Pinch of sea salt
- Pinch of fresh ground black pepper
- 1-2 tbsp. extra virgin olive oil
- 2 c. mixed greens of choice, chopped
- ½ c. radishes, trimmed, chopped
- ¼ c. celery, chopped
- 1 green onion (both white and green parts), chopped
- 1 red onion, chopped
- 2 tbsp. olive oil or preferred vegan dressing

Directions

1. Preheat grill to medium-high heat.

2. Cut any excess/visible fat from the chicken breasts, and rinse the chicken breasts in cool running water; pat dry with paper towels. Sprinkle with sea salt, black pepper, and drizzle on the olive oil. Grill chicken for 5-6 minutes per side or until cooked through and juices run clear. Transfer to a cutting board, let rest 3-5 minutes, then chop.

3. While the chicken is grilling, prepare the other ingredients as directed. In a large salad bowl, combine the chopped grilled chicken, chopped greens, and chopped veggies. Toss/stir to combine.

4. Drizzle on olive oil or preferred vegan dressing. Toss to coat. Transfer salad to a serving dish, serve and enjoy!

Nutritional Data

Calories: 392
Total Fat: 18
Carbohydrates: 17
Fiber: 5
Protein: 37

●●●

VEGETABLE KABOBS WITH PESTO

To be served with pre-cooked chargrilled chicken.

Servings: 1-2 (Serving Size: 3 vegetable kabobs with ½ c. pesto)
Total Time – Prep to Finish: 30 minutes

Ingredients

- ½ eggplant, cut into chunks
- ½-1 zucchini, cut into chunks,
- 1 bell pepper, cut into chunks
- 9 pints cherry tomatoes
- 1 red onion, cut into quarters
- ½-1 c. preferred pesto, divided
- 3-6 bamboo skewers (presoaked in water for 20 minutes.)

Directions

1. Place the bamboo skewers in cool water to soak for 20 minutes.
2. Prepare vegetables as directed.
3. Preheat the grill to medium-high heat.
4. Place the veggies in a large bowl. Pour ½ c. of the pesto into the bowl over the vegetables, and toss until the vegetables are completely coated.
5. Skewer the vegetables in desired order onto each bamboo skewer, and grill for 5-7 minutes, turning as needed, until the veggies are lightly charred and fork tender.
6. Place 3 veggie kabobs on a serving dish alongside the remaining ½ c. pesto, to serve. Freeze any remaining kabobs to be used as desired)

Nutritional Data

Calories: 331
Total Fat: 16
Carbohydrates: 38
Fiber: 18
Protein: 22

•••

VEGETABLE RATATOUILLE

Servings: 4 (Serving Size: 1½ - 2 cups)
Total Time – Prep to Finish: 10 minutes

Ingredients

- 3 tbsp. coconut oil
- 3 red bell peppers, thinly sliced
- 3 cloves garlic, crushed
- 1 eggplants, chopped
- 3 zucchini, sliced diagonally
- 1½ tbsp. red wine vinegar
- 2-3 large tomatoes, chopped
- ¾ c. cold water
- Sea salt, to taste
- Fresh ground black pepper, to taste

Directions

1. Place the coconut oil in a Dutch oven or a large, heavy-bottomed saucepan. Let the oil heat up over

medium-high heat. Add in the red bell pepper and onion. Sauté for 2 minutes or until softened.

2. While the pepper/onion is sautéing, chop up the eggplant, and slice the zucchini, diagonally, into rounds. Add the eggplant and zucchini to the pepper/onion, and stir to combine. Let sauté for 2 more minutes or just until just softened.

3. Next, add in the vinegar and chopped tomato. Cook for 30 seconds, stirring constantly, until the vinegar has evaporated. Add in ¼ c. cold water, season with salt and black pepper and bring to a simmer. Allow the ratatouille to simmer, covered, for 4 minutes or until the sauce has thickened and the vegetables are fork-tender.

4. Place 2 cups ratatouille on each serving plate and enjoy!

Nutritional Data

Calories: 194
Total Fat: 11
Carbohydrates: 22
Fiber: 10
Protein: 5

•••

TURKEY CHEESE BURGER ON BIBB LETTUCE

Servings: 4 (Serving Size: 1 turkey burger)
Total Time – Prep to Finish: 15 minutes

Ingredients

- 1-lb. organic ground turkey
- Pinch of sea salt, or to taste
- Pinch of fresh ground black pepper, or to taste
- Pinch of crushed red pepper flakes, or to taste
- 4 slices raw cheese of choice
- 1-2 large Bibb lettuce leaves per burger patty
- 1 avocado, peeled, stone removed/discarded and the flesh sliced (opt.)

Directions

1. Form the turkey into 4 patties. Sprinkle with the sea salt, black pepper, and crushed red pepper flakes.

2. Place a large skillet over medium heat. Add in the turkey burger patties and cook for 5-7 minutes per side or until the sides are nicely browned and the patties are cooked through.

3. Place a slice of raw cheese over each patty and cook for 1-2 minutes more or just until the cheese begins to melt.

4. Lay 2 slices of Bibb lettuce on a serving plate. Transfer the turkey burger on top of the lettuce and top with the sliced avocado, if using. Serve and enjoy!

Nutritional Data

Calories: 434
Total Fat: 31

Carbohydrates: 5
Fiber: 4
Protein: 39

•••

CUCUMBER AND APPLE SALAD WITH CHARGRILLED CHICKEN

Servings: 1 (Serving Size: 2 c. salad with 4-6 oz. chicken)
Total Time – Prep to Finish: 10 minutes

Ingredients

- Leftover (4-6 oz.) chargrilled chicken from previous night's dinner, reheated and sliced into cubes
- ½ medium Granny Smith apple, chopped
- ½ c. cucumber, chopped
- 2 c. green leaf lettuce, chopped
- 2 tbsp. extra-virgin olive oil
- 2 tbsp. balsamic vinegar

Directions

1. Prepare ingredients as directed.

2. Reheat the chicken in either the microwave or in a skillet for 2-4 minutes (depending on method) or until heated through. Transfer to a cutting board, and cut the reheated chargrilled chicken into cubes.

3. In a salad bowl, combine the chicken, green leaf lettuce, chopped apple, and chopped cucumber. Toss/stir to mix well.

4. Drizzle on the oil and vinegar. Toss to mix well.

5. Transfer to a serving plate and enjoy!

Nutritional Data

Calories: 457
Total Fat: 31
Carbohydrates: 18
Fiber: 12
Protein: 27

●●●

CHARGRILLED CHICKEN, BLACKBERRY AND BABY ARUGULA SALAD

Cost Conscious Meal: A pint of mixed berries and a bag of mixed greens costs less than $5 dollars and can be divided and spread out to make smoothies, simple salads, sandwiches/wraps, and more!

Servings: 2 (Serving Size: 2 c. salad)
Total Time – Prep to Finish: 10 minutes

Ingredients

- Leftover (4-6 oz.) chargrilled chicken from previous night's dinner, reheated and sliced into cubes

- 1 c. fresh blackberries
- 2 c. baby arugula, chopped
- 2 tbsp. lemon juice per salad
- 2 tbsp. balsamic vinegar per salad

Directions

1. Prepare ingredients as directed.

2. Reheat the chicken in either the microwave or in a skillet for 2-4 minutes (depending on method) or until heated through. Transfer to a cutting board, and cut the reheated chargrilled chicken into cubes.

3. In a salad bowl, combine 2 c. baby arugula and 1 c. fresh blackberries.

4. Drizzle on the 2 tbsp. lemon juice and 2 tbsp. vinegar and toss to blend salad contents.

5. Transfer to a serving dish and enjoy.

6. Store the remaining baby arugula and blackberries in sealable stay-fresh containers, and place in the refrigerator to be used as directed throughout the 30-day meal plan. When ready to serve, just remove from refrigerator, toss/stir to revive the salad, add on the lemon juice and vinegar, then enjoy!

Nutritional Data

Calories: 212
Total Fat: 4
Carbohydrates 15

Fiber: 8

Protein: 29

•••

GRILLED SALMON SALAD WITH BLUEBERRIES AND MINT

Servings: 1 (Serving Size: 2 cups salad; 4-6 oz. grilled salmon)
Total Time – Prep to Finish: 20 minutes

Ingredients

- 4-6 ounces leftover wild caught grilled salmon from previous night's dinner, (reheated, if desired) and broken into bite-size pieces.
- 2 c. baby spinach, chopped or torn
- ½ c. fresh blueberries
- 1-2 tbsp. fresh mint, torn
- Juice from 1 lemon
- 2 tbsp. extra virgin olive oil

Directions

1. Reheat the salmon, if desired, or serve it chilled. Break the salmon into bite-size pieces.
2. In a salad bowl, combine the baby spinach, blueberries, and fresh mint. Toss to mix.
3. Drizzle on the olive oil and toss again to blend salad contents.

4. Transfer salad to a serving dish, arrange the pieces of grilled salmon over the salad, and then drizzle the lemon juice over the salmon and salad. Enjoy!

Nutritional Data

Calories: 408
Total Fat: 30
Carbohydrates: 13
Fiber: 4
Protein: 26

●●●

KALE, ARUGULA, AND SPICED STEAK SALAD

Servings: 1 (Serving Size: 2 c. salad; 4-6 oz. steak; 1/8-1/4 c. dressing)
Total Time – Prep to Finish: 20 minutes

Ingredients

- Leftover (4-6 oz.) Spiced Steak from previous night's dinner, reheated and sliced into thin strips
- ½ c. baby kale, stems removed, chopped; divided
- 1½ c. baby arugula, chopped
- 3 cherry tomatoes, sliced
- 1-2 tbsp. extra-virgin olive oil
- 1-2 tbsp. balsamic vinegar per salad

Directions

1. Wash and prepare the salad ingredients as directed.

2. Reheat the steak strips either in the microwave or in a skillet for 2-4 minutes (depending on method) or until heated through. Transfer to a cutting board, and slice the steak into thin strips.

3. In a salad bowl, toss together ½ c. of the chopped baby kale, 1½ c. baby arugula, and 2 sliced cherry tomatoes. Drizzle 1-2 tbsp. each of the olive oil and balsamic vinegar over the salad contents, and sprinkle in a pinch of sea salt and black pepper, if desired. Then toss to mix.

4. Transfer salad to a serving dish; arrange the 4-6 oz. of the steak strips over the salad, then serve and enjoy.

Nutritional Data

Calories: 363
Total Fat: 18
Carbohydrates: 24
Fiber: 6
Protein: 31

●●●

SPINACH AND TOASTED WALNUT SALAD WITH BAKED CHICKEN

Servings: 1 (Serving Size: 2 c. salad; 4-6 oz. baked chicken breast
Total Time – Prep to Finish: 10 minutes

Ingredients

- 4-6 oz. leftover baked chicken breast, reheated
- 2 c. baby spinach
- 1/8 c. walnuts, chopped coarsely
- 2 tbsp. extra-virgin olive oil
- 1 tbsp. balsamic vinegar
- 1/8 clove garlic, crushed
- 1/8 tsp. ground cinnamon (opt.)

Directions

1. Reheat the leftover baked chicken breast in the oven or microwave. Time varies depending on method: 1½-3 minutes in microwave on high (100%) power OR 10-15 minutes in the oven at 350°F or until heated through.

2. Meanwhile, place a small skillet over medium-low heat. Drop in the chopped walnuts and stir constantly for 3-5 minutes or until the walnuts are nicely (lightly) toasted.

3. Next, combine the olive oil, vinegar, crushed garlic, and cinnamon (if using) in a small bowl and whisk to blend well.

4. Place the spinach and toasted walnuts in a salad bowl and toss/stir to mix. Drizzle the dressing over the surface of the salad, and toss to incorporate.

5. Transfer the salad to a serving dish, serve alongside the chargrilled chicken breast and enjoy!

•••

MIXED GREENS AND TILAPIA SALAD WITH MACADAMIA NUTS

*Cost Conscious Meal: Combining a bag of mixed greens with leftover meat or fish can make an inexpensive, filling, salad that you can enjoy at home, at work or on the go!

Servings: 1 (Serving Size: 2 c. salad with 4-6 oz. tilapia)
Total Time – Prep to Finish: 10 minutes

Ingredients

- Leftover (4-6 oz.) broiled tilapia from previous night's dinner, reheated and broken into bite-size pieces.
- 2 c. mixed greens of choice, chopped
- 1-2 tbsp. macadamia nuts, chopped
- 2 tbsp. extra virgin olive oil, for dressing

Directions

1. Reheat the tilapia in the microwave for 1-2 minutes or until heated through. Transfer to a cutting board, and break the fillet into smaller, bite-size pieces.
2. In a salad bowl, place the mixed greens. Arrange the pieces of tilapia over the greens.
3. Sprinkle the salad with the chopped macadamia nuts to garnish.
4. Finally, Drizzle the salad with the olive oil as a dressing and enjoy!

Nutritional Data

Calories: 407
Total Fat: 35
Carbohydrates: 3
Fiber: 2
Protein: 24

•••

CHARGRILLED CHICKEN SALAD WITH WHITE BEETS

Cost Conscious Meal: Adding leftover grilled chicken from dinner to liven up a simple salad makes for a fulfilling and super inexpensive lunch!

Servings: 1 (Serving Size: 4-6 oz. chicken; 2 c. salad)
Total Time – Prep to Finish: 15 minutes

Ingredients

- Leftover 4-6 oz. chargrilled chicken breast, reheated and cut into strips
- 2 c. romaine lettuce, chopped
- 3 cherry tomatoes, halved
- 1-2 white beets, sliced
- 2 tbsp. balsamic vinegar
- 2 tbsp. extra virgin olive oil (opt.)

Directions

1. Prepare ingredients as directed.

2. Reheat the chicken in either the microwave or in a skillet for 2-4 minutes (depending on method) or until heated through. Transfer to a cutting board, and cut the reheated chargrilled chicken into thin strips.

3. Meanwhile, in a large salad bowl, combine the romaine lettuce and halved cherry tomatoes. Toss to mix well. Drizzle the balsamic vinegar (and olive oil, if using) over the salad contents. Toss well to mix.

4. Transfer the salad to a serving dish and arrange 6 oz. of the chargrilled chicken breast strips over the salad and serve.

5. Place the remaining salad/chicken in a stay-fresh container, and store in the refrigerator, to be used as directed during the 30-day meal plan.

Nutritional Data

Calories: 468
Total Fat: 32
Carbohydrates: 18
Fiber: 5
Protein: 29

●●●

STRAWBERRY, ROMAINE, AND AVOCADO SALAD WITH SPICED STEAK STRIPS

Servings: 1 (Serving Size: 2 c. salad; 4-6 oz. steak)
Total Time – Prep to Finish: 10 minutes

Ingredients

- Leftover (4-6 oz.) Spiced Steak from previous night's dinner, reheated and sliced into thin strips
- 1 c. fresh strawberries, hulled and halved
- 2 c. romaine lettuce, chopped
- ¼-½ ripe avocado, peeled/stone removed; sliced
- 1-2 tbsp. toasted walnuts, chopped coarsely
- 2 tbsp. balsamic vinegar
- 2 tbsp. extra virgin olive oil

Directions

1. Wash and prepare the salad ingredients as directed.
2. Reheat the steak strips either in the microwave or in a skillet for 2-4 minutes (depending on method) or until heated through.

3. In a large salad bowl, combine the halved berries, chopped romaine, and toasted walnuts. Toss to mix.
4. Transfer 2 c. of the salad to a serving dish.
5. Drizzle on the oil and vinegar; toss to mix. Arrange the reheated steak strips and desired amount of sliced avocado over the salad, then serve and enjoy!

Nutritional Data

Calories: 395
Total Fat: 23
Carbohydrates: 9

Fiber: 4

Protein: 15

●●●

ITALIAN SAUTÉED FENNEL & RADICCHIO SALAD WITH GRILLED CHICKEN

Servings: 1 (Serving Size: 4-6 oz. grilled chicken strips; 1½ c. salad)
Total Time – Prep to Finish: 20 minutes

Ingredients

- ½-lb. fully-cooked grilled chicken breast strips, heated through

- 3-5 tbsp. red wine vinegar

- 2 small garlic cloves, finely chopped

- 1 large fennel bulb, sliced

- ½ tbsp. coconut oil

- 1-2 small heads of radicchio, sliced or chopped to yield 2 cups

- ¼ tsp. sea salt, divided, plus more to taste, if needed

- ½ tbsp. lemon juice

- 1-2 tsp. fresh tarragon leaves, torn, to garnish

Directions

1. Place the fully-cooked grilled chicken strips in a skillet over medium-high heat and cook 3-5 minutes

or until strips are heated through. Remove chicken from heat and set aside.

2. Wipe out the skillet and place it over medium heat. Add in ½ tbsp. coconut oil and allow it to heat up. Add in the chopped garlic; sauté 1-2 minutes or until fragrant. Add in the sliced fennel, season with 1 tsp. sea salt, or to taste. Sauté for 2-3 minutes or until the fennel is slightly softened.

3. Add in the sliced radicchio; season again with ½ tsp. sea salt, or to taste. Sauté 1-2 minutes more or until radicchio begins wilting and turning brown in spots. Remove from heat immediately and add a splash of lemon juice.

4. To serve, place the radicchio/fennel salad mixture on a serving plate and top the grilled chicken strips, and a few of the torn tarragon leaves. Finally, drizzle the salad with red wine vinegar; season with additional sea salt, if needed, to taste, then serve immediately.

Nutritional Data

Calories: 289
Total Fat: 7
Carbs: 27
Dietary Fiber: 7
Sugars: 7
Protein: 24

●●●

CHICKEN CURRY SOUP WITH COCONUT AND LIME

Servings: 1 (Serving Size: 1½ - 2 c. soup)
Total Time – Prep to Finish: 20 minutes

Ingredients

- 1 c. reduced-sodium chicken broth
- ¼ c. unsweetened coconut milk
- ¼ tbsp. curry powder
- ½ jalapeno pepper, seeded and minced
- 6-8 oz. boneless skinless chicken breast halves, cut into ¾-inch cubes
- 1 tbsp. fresh lime juice
- ¼ tsp. sea salt, or to taste
- ¼ tsp. fresh ground black pepper, or to taste
- ½ c. green onion (white and green parts), chopped
- ½ c. fresh cilantro, chopped
- 1 c. cauliflower, riced and steamed
- 2 lime wedges, to serve

Directions

1. First, rice the cauliflower and steam until tender and heated through.

2. Meanwhile, bring the chicken broth, coconut milk, curry powder and the jalapeno to a simmer in a heavy medium saucepan over medium heat.

3. Add chicken and simmer for about 5 minutes or until chicken is just cooked through, stirring frequently. Stir in the lime juice and season, to taste, with sea salt and fresh ground black pepper.

4. Place the cauliflower rice in a serving bowl. Ladle the soup over the rice.

5. To serve, garnish with chopped green onion and fresh cilantro. Season with additional salt and pepper, if needed, to taste and serve with 2 wedges of lime.

Nutritional Data

Calories: 236

Total Fat: 7

Carbs: 14

Dietary Fiber: 5

Sugars: 5

Protein: 28

chapter 9

DINNER RECIPES
BAKED CHICKEN AND SAUTÉED BRUSSELS SPROUTS

Servings: 2 (Serving Size: 6 oz. chicken; 1½ c. sautéed Brussels sprouts)
Total Time – Prep to Finish: 55 minutes

Ingredients

- 2 (4-6 oz.) free-range boneless, skinless chicken breasts
- 4 tbsp. extra-virgin olive oil, divided
- 2 tbsp. lemon juice, divided
- ½ tsp. salt, or to taste, divided
- ¼ tsp. fresh ground black pepper, divided
- 1/8-1/4 tsp. tarragon (opt.)
- 1 tsp. dried parsley, divided
- 4 c. small Brussels sprouts
- 1 tbsp. extra-virgin olive oil (plus more for rubbing)

- 1/8 tsp. fresh ground black pepper, or to taste
- ¼ tsp. sea salt, or to taste
- ¼ c. preferred raw cheese, finely grated

Directions

1. Preheat oven to 350°F. Rinse the chicken breasts in cool running water; cut off any visible excess fat, and place the chicken breasts in a baking dish. Season the chicken with sea salt, black pepper, and the tarragon (opt.). Drizzle ½ tbsp. lemon juice and ½ tbsp. olive oil over each chicken breast. Then top each breast with ½ tsp. dried parsley, and ½ tbsp. more of lemon juice.

2. Place the chicken in the preheated oven, and bake for 35-40 minutes or until the chicken is cooked through and juices run clear (the chicken should reach an internal temperature of 165°F).

3. When the chicken is nearly finished baking, prepare the Brussels sprouts. Wash the sprouts well, and remove and discard any outer leaves.

4. Slice each sprout in half lengthwise from the stem to the top of the sprout, then brush the halves with 3 tbsp. of the olive oil, or as needed.

5. Place a large sauté pan over medium heat. Add in the remaining 1 tbsp. olive oil, and allow it a couple of minutes to heat up just a little, then lay the Brussels sprouts in the pan, flat half facing down.

6. Sprinkle the sprouts with sea salt and black pepper. Allow the sprouts to sauté, moving the sprouts around, so they do no stick to the pan.

7. Sauté for 3-5 minutes or until the flat side of the sprouts turns lightly golden brown and are fork tender (make sure you can pierce the fork completely through the sprouts.

8. Once fork tender, turn up the heat to high, and cook for 2-4 minutes or just long enough for the flat sides of the sprouts to become caramelized and a deep golden brown. Then begin tossing/stirring and moving the sprouts around to gain a little bit of browning on the rounded sides as well.

9. Transfer 2 c. to a serving dish, and sprinkle on a bit more sea salt and black pepper, if needed, and then finally, sprinkle the finely raw grated cheese over the sprouts. Serve alongside the baked chicken and enjoy!

10. Let the remaining chicken and sprouts cool completely at room temperature. Then store in sealable containers in the refrigerator to serve as lunch the following day. When ready to serve, just remove from refrigerator and reheat!

Nutritional Data

Calories: 415
Total Fat: 44
Carbohydrates: 1
Fiber: 0
Protein: 7

●●●

SPICED STEAK AND GRILLED PEPPER SALAD

*Cost Conscious Meal: This dish costs less than $4.50 per serving; a dish originally prepared for lunch makes an excellent and very inexpensive side dish!

Servings: 4 (Serving Size: 1 (4-6 oz.) grilled sirloin steak; 1½ c. salad)Total Time – Prep to Finish: 35 minutes

Ingredients

- 6 (4-6 oz. each) grass-fed sirloin steaks (New York cut or preferred cut), all visible fat trimmed
- 2 2/3 tbsp. white wine vinegar
- 4 large garlic cloves, crushed
- 1 1/3 tbsp. water
- 1 1/3 tbsp. ground coriander
- 2 tsp. ground cumin
- 2 tsp. chili powder
- 4 bell peppers, (red, yellow, green, orange), stems/seeds discarded, halved
- ¼ c. black olives, pitted/halved cup halved and pitted oil-cured black olives
- ¼ c. sun-dried tomatoes, rinsed/chopped
- 1-2 tbsp. extra-virgin olive oil
- 1-2 tbsp. balsamic vinegar
- 1/8-1/4 tsp. sea salt, to taste

- 1/8-1/4 c. raw feta or goat cheese, crumbled

Directions

1. Use a sharp knife to very lightly score both sides of the steak in a diamond pattern. In a small bowl, combine the white wine vinegar with the garlic, water, coriander, cumin, and chili powder, and mix well. Use a pastry brush to brush the mixture evenly over both sides of each steak. Place steaks on a plate, covered, in the fridge for 15 minutes to marinate.

2. Preheat a barbecue grill on medium-high. Place the bell pepper halves, face down, on the grill, and cook for 4-5 minutes or until nicely charred. Turn the peppers over, and continue grilling for 4-5 minutes more or until the peppers are nicely charred. Remove from grill, and transfer to a cutting board.

3. Next, place the steaks on the grill, and cook for 5-7 minutes per side for medium or until cooked to your liking. While the steaks are grilling, prepare the side salad.

4. First, when the grilled peppers are cool enough to handle, chop them up into bite-sized pieces. Place the chopped bell peppers in a large salad bowl. Add in the halved olives, chopped sun-dried tomatoes, olive oil, vinegar, sea salt, and raw crumbled cheese, and toss/stir to mix well.

5. Serve one of the steaks alongside 1½ c. of the grilled pepper salad. Reserve the remaining steaks and salad to be used as directed throughout the 30-day meal plan.

Nutritional Data

Calories: 355
Total Fat: 18
Carbohydrates: 10
Fiber: 4
Protein: 37

•••

STEAK AND ASPARAGUS STIR-FRY

Servings: 4 (Serving Size: (2 c. stir-fry)
Total Time – Prep to Finish: 20 minutes

Ingredients

- 2 tbsp. coconut oil
- 2-lb. asparagus, trimmed and cut diagonally into 1½-inch lengths, to yield 8 c.
- 4 (4-6 oz. each) grass-fed steaks (preferred cut), grilled and sliced into thin strips
- 2-3 tsp. fresh ginger, peeled and finely chopped
- 4 small cloves of garlic, minced
- 4 green onions (white and green parts), sliced, divided
- 4 tbsp. sesame seeds, toasted, to garnish (opt.)

Directions

1. Bring a Dutch oven or large stock pot of water to a boil. While waiting for water to boil, prepare the ingredients as directed. When water begins to boil,

add the 8 c. of asparagus pieces and parboil for 2 minutes, then drain and rinse in cold water. Drain again, and set aside.

2. Place a wok over medium-high heat. Add in 1 tbsp. coconut oil, and allow it to heat up. Add the asparagus and stir-fry in for about 2 minutes or until lightly browned. Remove asparagus from wok; set aside.

3. Add another 1 tbsp. coconut oil to wok. Let it heat. Then add in the steak strips in a single layer, followed by the chopped ginger, minced garlic, and green onions. Stir to mix well. Stir-fry for 5-7 minutes or until the steak is cooked through. Return the asparagus to the wok, and toss to mix with other ingredients.

4. Transfer 2 c. the stir-fry to a serving dish and garnish with 1 tbsp. toasted sesame seeds, if desired, and then serve and enjoy!

5. Divide the remaining 6 c. steak-asparagus stir-fry into 2 cup portions in separate sealable containers, and store in the freezer to be used as directed throughout the 30-day meal plan. When ready to use, just reheat and serve!

Nutritional Data

Calories: 296
Total Fat: 15
Carbohydrates: 13
Fiber: 6
Protein: 33

●●●

GRILLED SALMON, ZUCCHINI, & BROCCOLI SALAD

Servings: 4 (Serving Size: 1 (6 oz.) salmon portion; 2 spears zucchini; 1½ c. salad)

Total Time – Prep to Finish: 30 minutes

Ingredients

- 2 large zucchini, thinly sliced (to yield 2 cups)
- 3 tbsp. extra-virgin olive oil, divided
- ½ tsp. sea salt, or to taste, divided
- ¼ tsp. fresh ground black pepper, or to taste
- ½ clove garlic, minced
- 2 (6 oz.) wild salmon fillets
- 1 tbsp. fresh basil, chopped
- 2/3 c. raw feta cheese, crumbled
- ½ c. organic whole or goat's milk plain yogurt
- 2 tbsp. lemon juice
- 2 cloves garlic, minced
- ½ tsp. fresh ground black pepper
- 6 c. broccoli florets, trimmed/chopped
- 1-2 cans gluten-free chickpeas, rinsed and drained
- 1 c. red bell pepper, chopped

Directions

1. Preheat grill to medium-high heat.

2. Place the sliced zucchini in a bowl with 2 tbsp. olive oil (or more as needed to evenly coat), ¼ tsp. sea salt, and ¼ tsp. black pepper. Toss to coat the zucchini in the oil and seasonings.

3. Mash the minced garlic and ¼ tsp. of the salt on a cutting board with the side of a chef's knife or a spoon until a paste forms. Transfer to a small bowl, and stir in the remaining 1 tbsp. olive oil.

4. Check the salmon for any pin bones; remove and discard. Measure out a piece of heavy-duty aluminum foil (or a double layer of regular foil) large enough for each salmon fillet. Coat the foil with cooking spray. Place the salmon skin-side-down on each piece of foil, and spread the garlic mixture all over it. Sprinkle each salmon fillet with up the fresh basil.

5. Transfer the salmon fillets on the foils to the grill. Grill for 10-12 minutes or until the salmon flakes easily and reaches an internal temperature of 145°F.

6. While the salmon is grilling, prepare the broccoli salad. In a large-sized mixing bowl, combine the raw crumbled cheese, the yogurt, minced garlic, lemon juice, and the black pepper. Whisk until smooth and well blended. Prepare the broccoli and bell pepper as directed, Then add them to the yogurt dressing, along with the rinsed/drained chickpeas. Toss/stir to mix, and coat the salad contents well with the yogurt dressing. Salad can be served chilled or at room temperature.

7. Using two large spatulas, slide one of the salmon fillets onto a serving plate, and serve alongside 2 spears of zucchini and the broccoli salad.

8. Store the remaining salmon fillets/zucchini/broccoli salad in the refrigerator/freezer in sealable containers to be used as directed throughout 30-day meal plan.

9. To grill the zucchini, place the slices directly on the grill. Let grill for 5-6 minutes, and then flip the slices and grill for an additional 5-6 minutes or until fork-tender. If you want crisscross grill marks, rotate each piece halfway through cooking on both sides.

10. To serve, place the remaining salmon fillet on a serving plate alongside 1½-2 c. of the grilled zucchini slices. Sprinkle the salmon fillet with a little of the remaining basil and serve.

Nutritional Data

Calories: 415
Total Fat: 20
Carbohydrates: 29
Fiber: 9
Protein: 33

●●●

CHARGRILLED CHICKEN AND ROASTED BROCCOLI AND BABY SPINACH SALAD

Cost Conscious Meal: This dish costs less than $3.75 per serving when using the grill and combining with fresh vegetables such as broccoli, asparagus, Brussels sprouts, fresh greens, etc.

Servings: 2 (Serving Size: 6 oz. chicken; 2 cups broccoli) – PLUS 6 extra breasts are grilled to store and use for other meals on the 30-day meal plan)

Total Time – Prep to Finish: 15 minutes

Ingredients

- 8 (6 oz. each) free-range boneless, skinless chicken breasts
- Zest from 1 lime, finely grated
- Juice from 4-6 limes
- 2 tbsp. plus 2 tbsp. extra virgin olive oil, divided
- 3 cloves garlic, crushed
- 2 c. roasted broccoli
- 2 tbsp. extra virgin olive oil, as needed
- 1/8-¼ tsp. sea salt
- 1/8 tsp. fresh ground black pepper
- 1½ c. baby spinach, torn
- ¼ c. cucumber, sliced
- 1/8 c. red onion, chopped
- 2 tbsp. vegan dressing of choice

Directions

1. Begin by roasting the broccoli: Preheat the oven to 425°F. Line a rimmed baking sheet with aluminum foil.

2. Place the broccoli on the foil-lined baking sheet. Drizzle with 2 tbsp. of the olive oil, and then sprinkle on the sea salt and black pepper.

3. Place in the middle of the preheated oven, and roast for 40-45 minutes or until the stems of the broccoli are fork tender. Toward the last 10 minutes or so, keep a watchful eye on the roasting broccoli as the florets can go from perfectly browned to black in a matter of a few minutes.

4. As soon as the broccoli is put in the oven to roast, begin grilling the chicken breasts as you have to account for marinating time. Cut any excess/visible fat from the chicken breasts, and rinse the chicken breasts in cool running water. Pat dry with paper towels.

5. Prepare the marinade by combining the lime zest, lime juice, the remaining ½ c. olive oil, and the crushed garlic into a shallow glass bowl. Whisk until the contents are well incorporated, adding a little more olive oil, if needed.

6. Place the chicken breasts in the marinade, turning to coat each breast with the marinade as best as possible – Cover the bowl with plastic wrap, and place in the refrigerator for at least 15 minutes to marinate. TIP: You could also combine the marinade in a doubled gallon-sized Ziploc bag, and place the chicken breasts

in the bag to marinate. Doing this can often make it easier to coat each piece with the marinade. If you are worried about the bag leaking, just lay the bag in a large bowl or in a shallow dish such as a pie pan to catch any leakage.

7. Preheat the grill. Place the chicken breasts on the grill, and grill for about 4-5 minutes per side or until nicely charred and cooked through. The chicken should reach an internal temperature of 165°F.

8. Remove the chicken from the grill, and allow to cool for 5 minutes.

9. Place one of the chargrilled breasts on a serving plate alongside the 2 c. of the roasted broccoli. Serve immediately.

10. For the remaining 7 chicken breasts: Place one of the breasts in a storage container, and store in the refrigerator to be used for the next day's lunch. Place the remaining 6 chargrilled chicken breasts in freezer wrap/freezer safe containers – individually – to be pulled out and reheated as directed throughout the 30-day meal plan. Allow the chicken breasts to cool completely at room temperature before placing in the freezer.

Nutritional Data

Calories: 391
Total Fat: 30
Carbohydrates: 17
Fiber: 5
Protein: 19

●●●

BAKED BASIL CHICKEN OVER FRESH GREENS WITH ASPARAGUS

Servings: 2 (Serving Size: 4-6 oz. baked chicken; 1 ½ c. fresh greens)Total Time – Prep to Finish: 45 minutes

Ingredients

- 2 (¾-lbs./approx. 4-6 oz. each) boneless, skinless chicken breast halves
- 1-lb asparagus spears
- 2 green onions (both white and green parts), chopped
- 1/8 c. extra-virgin olive oil
- 1 tbsp. white wine vinegar
- 1 tsp. fresh ginger, chopped fine
- 1 tbsp. fresh basil, chopped fine (or 1-2 tsp. dried basil)
- 3 c. fresh spinach (or fresh greens of choice)

Directions

1. Rinse the chicken breasts in cool, running water; pat dry using paper towel. Cut away any visible or excess fat.

2. In a medium-size glass bowl, combine the green onion, olive oil, vinegar, fresh ginger, and fresh (or dried) basil; whisk together to create the marinade.

3. Arrange the chicken breasts in a shallow baking dish, and pour the marinade over the chicken, turning to coat. Cover with plastic wrap, and place the marinating chicken in the refrigerator for 30 minutes.

4. Preheat oven to 375°F. Line a rimmed baking sheet with aluminum foil. Place the chicken breasts on the foil-lined baking sheet, and arrange the rinsed/dried asparagus spears around the chicken breasts. Place the baking sheet in the preheated oven. Bake the chicken/asparagus for 35-45 minutes or until the asparagus is fork tender and the chicken breasts are cooked through and juices run clear.

5. To serve, place a baked chicken breast on each plate, and serve with over a bed of fresh spinach or preferred greens and serve alongside 3-4 spears of asparagus.

6. Store the remaining Chicken/Greens/Asparagus in the sealable containers to be used for lunch the following day.

Nutritional Data

Calories: 488
Total Fat: 29
Carbohydrates: 25
Fiber: 13
Protein: 39

●●●

BROILED TILAPIA AND STEAMED VEGGIES

Servings: 3 (Serving Size: 1 (4 to 6 oz.) tilapia fillet; 1½-2 c. vegetables of choice)

Total Time – Prep to Finish: 20 minutes

Ingredients

- 3 (4-6 oz.) wild caught tilapia fillets
- sea salt, to taste
- fresh ground black pepper, or to taste
- 1 tsp. dried oregano
- 1 tsp. dried parsley
- 3 tsp. extra-virgin olive oil, divided
- 1 clove fresh garlic, minced
- 1½-2 c. steamed or roasted vegetables of choice per serving

Directions

1. To prepare, turn on the broiler to low and preheat. Align an oven rack in the upper half of the oven about 8 inched from the broiler flame. Line a broiler pan with aluminum foil.

2. Rinse the tilapia fillets and pat dry. Then lay the tilapia on the foil-lined broiler pan, and season the fillets with the sea salt and black pepper, to taste, followed by the dried oregano and dried parsley.

3. Drizzle each fillet with 1 tsp. olive oil, and then sprinkle on a pinch of the fresh minced garlic.

4. Place the broiler pan holding the tilapia fillets in the oven, and cook for 5-7 minutes or until the fish is cooked through.

5. Remove from broiler, and immediately splash the fillets with lemon juice.

6. Transfer one of the tilapia fillets to a serving dish, and serve alongside steamed or roasted vegetables of choice.

7. Store the remaining fillets individually in freezer wrap, and store the wrapped fillets in the freezer to be used as directed throughout the 30-day meal plan.

Nutritional Data

Calories: 194
Total Fat: 6
Carbohydrates: 4
Fiber: 2
Protein: 31

●●●

BARBECUED SIRLOIN IN DIJON DRESSING WITH GRILLED VEGETABLES

Servings: 4 (Serving Size: 1 (4-6 oz.) sirloin steak; ¼ c. Dijon dressing; 2 c. grilled mixed vegetables)

Total Time – Prep to Finish: 30 minutes

Ingredients

- 4 (4-6 oz.) grass-fed beef sirloin steaks

- 2 tbsp. fresh basil, coarsely chopped
- 2 tsp. fresh ground black pepper
- 2 tbsp. Dijon mustard
- 2 tbsp. beef broth
- 2 tbsp. white wine vinegar
- 8 c. grilled mixed vegetables

Directions

1. In a bowl, combine the basil, the black pepper, the olive oil, the Dijon mustard and the white wine vinegar.

2. Rub the marinade onto the sirloin steaks, and refrigerate for at least 15 minutes to marinate.

3. Preheat the grill to medium-high, and cook the steak 5-7 minutes per side or until desired doneness is reached. Meanwhile, grill chosen vegetables until heated through.

4. Let the meat rest around 5-10 minutes before serving. Serve alongside 2 c. grilled vegetables.

Nutritional Data

Calories: 353
Total Fat: 6
Carbohydrates: 39
Fiber: 20
Protein: 36

●●●

BLACK BEAN CHILI

Servings: 8 (Serving Size: 1 ½-2 c. chili)
Total Time – Prep to Finish: 30 minutes

Ingredients

- 2-lbs. organic ground turkey (or grass-fed ground beef, if preferred)
- 2-3 cans gluten-free black beans, rinsed/drained
- 1 large white onion(s), diced
- 1 green bell pepper, chopped (opt,)
- 3-4 (14-oz.) cans diced tomatoes
- ½ c. water
- 2-4 tbsp. chili powder, to taste
- Desired toppings: raw shredded cheese, sliced green onions, etc.

Directions

1. Place a Dutch oven or a deep, heavy-bottomed pan over medium heat. Add in the ground turkey (or beef) and cook, stirring occasionally to help crumble up the meat for 6-8 minutes or until browned. Drain, then return meat to the Dutch oven/pan.

2. Add in the onion and bell pepper, and cook for 2-3 minutes, mixing the veggies with the ground meat, until the onion and pepper are fork tender. Sprinkle in the desired amount of chili powder; stir to incorporate.

3. Next, add in the water, black beans, and diced tomatoes, and stir to incorporate. Then allow the contents to come to a boil, stirring occasionally. Once the chili begins to boil, reduce heat to low, cover and simmer for 20 minutes, stirring occasionally. Then uncover and continue cooking an additional 5 minutes more.

4. Ladle 1 ½-2 c. of chili into a bowl, top with desired toppings, and enjoy.

5. Let the remaining chili cool completely. Then using sealable storage containers, store the remaining chili in separate 1½-2 cup portions to be pulled out and reheated as directed throughout 30-day meal plan.

Nutritional Data

Calories: 350
Total Fat: 14
Carbohydrates: 21
Fiber: 7
Protein: 39

●●●

MEDITERRANEAN STEW

Servings: 8 (Serving Size: (1½ - 2 c. stew)
Total Time – Prep to Finish: 20 minutes

Ingredients

- 2-lbs. grass-fed beef sirloin, cut into 1-inch pieces (or use precut stew meat).

- 1-2 tbsp. coconut oil

- 1 c. button mushrooms, sliced
- 1 c. frozen pearl onions, thawed
- 4 cloves garlic, minced
- 3½ c. beef broth or stock, divided
- 3 (28 oz.) cans crushed tomatoes with juice
- 3 (6 oz.) cans tomato paste
- 1 tbsp. arrowroot powder
- 2 c. baby spinach, torn
- 1/8-1/4 c. fresh basil, chopped
- 1/8-1/4 c. fresh oregano, chopped
- 1 tbsp. sea salt, or to taste
- 1 tbsp. fresh ground black pepper, or to taste

Directions

1. Begin by preparing the beef, trim off any excess fat, and cut into 1-inch pieces. Season with sea salt and pepper. Place a Dutch oven or large pot over medium-high heat. Add in 1 tbsp. coconut oil, and let it heat up. Add the pieces of beef to the skillet, and brown it on all sides for 5 to 7 minutes. Transfer to plate, and set aside until needed.

2. In the Dutch oven/pot, now add in ½ tbsp. coconut oil, and let melt; then combine the sliced button mushrooms, pearl onions, and garlic, and sauté for 5 minutes, stirring often. Place the browned meat back into the Dutch oven/pot, and stir to combine the contents. Add in 3 c. beef broth (or stock), cans

of crushed tomatoes (plus juices), tomato paste, and a little water, if needed, to thin. Bring contents to a boil. Then reduce heat to medium, cover and simmer for 45 minutes.

3. In a small bowl, whisk together the remaining ¼ tsp. broth (or stock) and 2 tbsp. arrowroot powder until the powder is dissolved. Then stir the mixture into the stew after 45 minutes, along with adding in the baby spinach, fresh basil, and the fresh oregano. Stir with wooden spoon to mix well. Sprinkle in the sea salt and black pepper, and stir to incorporate.

4. Cook for an additional 20-30 minutes or until the beef is cooked through, the onions are fork tender, and the spinach is nicely wilted. Taste, and adjust seasonings as necessary. Note: You can also make this stew by combining all ingredients into a slow cooker, and cooking on LOW heat for 7 hours or on HIGH heat for 3-4 hours.

5. Ladle 1½-2 c. stew per serving bowl, and serve. Let the remaining stew cool completely. Then using sealable storage containers, store the remaining stew in separate 1½-2 cup portions to be pulled out and reheated as directed throughout 30-day meal plan.

Nutritional Data

Calories: 329
Total Fat: 6
Carbohydrates: 40
Fiber: 8
Protein: 37

•••

EGGPLANT RATATOUILLE

Servings: 1 (Serving Size: 1½ - 2 cups)
Total Time – Prep to Finish: 10 minutes

Ingredients

- ½ tbsp. coconut oil
- ½ red bell pepper, thinly sliced
- 1 clove garlic, crushed
- ¼ small eggplant, chopped
- ½ small zucchini, sliced diagonally
- 1½ tbsp. red wine vinegar
- ½ large tomatoes, chopped
- ¼ c. cold water
- ¼ tsp. sea salt, to taste
- 1/8 tsp. fresh ground black pepper, to taste

Directions

1. Place the coconut oil in a Dutch oven or a large, heavy-bottomed saucepan. Let the oil heat up over medium-high heat. Add in the red bell pepper and onion. Sauté for 2 minutes or until softened.

2. While the pepper/onion is sautéing, chop up the eggplant and slice the zucchini, diagonally, into rounds. Add the eggplant and zucchini to the pepper/

onion and stir to combine. Let sauté for 2 more minutes or just until just softened.

3. Next, add in the vinegar and chopped tomato. Cook for 30 seconds, stirring constantly, until the vinegar has evaporated. Add in ¼ c. cold water, season with salt and black pepper and bring to a simmer. Allow the ratatouille to simmer, covered, for 4 minutes or until the sauce has thickened and the vegetables are fork-tender.

4. Place 1½-2 cups ratatouille on a serving plate and enjoy!

Nutritional Data

Calories: 147

Total Fat: 12

Carbohydrates: 11

Fiber: 2

Sugars: 3

Protein: 4

chapter 10

SNACK AND DESSERT RECIPES

SNACK/DESSERT RECIPE: CHOCOLATE-AVOCADO BROWNIES WITH WALNUTS

Servings: 12 – Yield: 12 Brownies (Serving Size: 1 brownie)
Total Time – Prep to Finish: 30

Ingredients

- ¾ c. almond meal
- ¼ c. unsweetened cocoa powder
- ½ tsp. baking powder
- ½ tsp. sea salt
- 3 tbsp. coconut oil
- 1 tsp. vanilla extract
- 2 large pasture-raised eggs
- 2 large ripe avocados

- 8 oz. vegan/allergen-free dark chocolate (70% or higher), chopped (such as Enjoy Life, Alter Eco, Kallari, etc.)
- 1 tbsp. Stevia powder extract (or 18-24 Stevia packets), or to taste
- ½ c. walnuts, chopped

Directions

1. Preheat oven to 350°F. Line an 8 x 8-inch baking pan with aluminum foil – enough so that the foil hangs over the sides of the pan. The overhanging foil will later act as handles, making it much easier to remove the brownies from the pan, in order to cut them.

2. Place the chopped chocolate and coconut oil in a microwave-safe bowl and heat in 15-30 second intervals, stirring between each interval with a wooden spoon, until the coconut oil and chocolate are completely melted and smooth. Stir the mixture well to blend. Let the coconut oil-chocolate mixture rest at room temperature for 5 minutes.

3. Meanwhile, peel the avocados, remove/discard stones, and place the avocado flesh in a large mixing bowl. Mash the avocado until the smooth. Next, stir the coconut oil-chocolate mixture in with the mashed avocado, and stir to blend. Next, stir in the Stevia powder extract (or packets) until completely incorporated. Then add the eggs – one at a time – then finally, stir in the vanilla extract.

4. In a separate bowl, first sift in the cocoa powder. Then stir in the almond meal, sea salt, and baking powder. Then add the dry mixture to the avocado mixture, and stir with a wooden spoon just until combined. Be sure to not over-mix. Fold in the walnuts, and then add the brownie batter to the prepared baking pan, and spread out to fill the pan, smoothing the top of the batter with a rubber spatula.

5. Place the pan in the preheated oven, and bake for 25-28 minutes or until a toothpick inserted into the center of the brownies comes out clean. Remove from oven, and let the brownies cool in the pan for 10 minutes. Then, holding the foil on either side of the pan, carefully lift the brownies out of the pan. Transfer the foil to a wire cooling rack, and allow the brownies to cool some more before slicing and serving. Store the remaining brownies in an airtight container at room temperature (or in the refrigerator) until needed as directed throughout the 30-day meal plan.

Nutritional Data

Calories: 298
Total Fat: 25
Carbohydrates: 25
Fiber: 1
Protein: 21

•••

SNACK/DESSERT RECIPE: GOOEY CHOCOLATE CHIP COOKIES

Cost Conscious Meal: This recipe makes 3 dozen cookies for less than $5 as it uses many ingredients from other week TWO meals – you can store them in the freezer until ready to serve.

Servings: 18 - Yield: 36 cookies (Serving Size: 2 cookies)
Total Time – Prep to Finish: 45 minutes

Ingredients

- 3 c. blanched almond flour
- 1 tbsp. coconut flour
- 1 tsp. sea salt
- ¾ tsp. baking soda
- ½ tsp. baking powder
- ½ c. grass-fed butter, melted
- ¼ tbsp. Stevia powder extract (or 8-10 Stevia packets)
- 1 tsp. agave nectar
- 2 large pasture-raised eggs, room temperature
- 1½ tbsp. pure vanilla extract
- 1 (10 oz.) package vegan semi-sweet chocolate chips (such as Enjoy Life or preferred brand)

Directions

1. To begin, combine the blanched almond flour, coconut flour, salt, baking soda, and baking powder and whisk until well blended; set aside.

2. In a food processor, combine the melted grass-fed butter and Stevia. Process mixture for 1 minute or

until the contents are blended well. Next, add in with the butter mixture, the agave nectar, the eggs, and the vanilla extract. Process until smooth and creamy. Add the wet ingredient to the flour mixture, and process in food processor, until the dough is completely blended and smooth.

3. Transfer the dough to a mixing bowl, and then fold in the chocolate chips, using a wooden spoon. When the chocolate chips are well incorporated, set the cookie dough aside to rest, at room temperature, for 15 minutes. The dough will become more solid and easier to work with as it rests.

4. Preheat the oven to 350°. Arrange the oven racks in center of oven. Line 2-3 baking sheets with parchment paper. Using a tablespoon, scoop out a rounded tablespoon of the dough, and drop it onto the parchment-lined baking sheet. Repeat until all the dough has been used up, placing them about 1-2 inches apart on the baking sheets. You should yield about 36 cookies.

5. Place the cookies in the oven, and bake for 10-12 minutes or until the edges/bottom of the cookies are golden brown and the centers appear slightly uncooked, puffy, and lightly crackled. Be careful not to let the cookies bake for more than 12 minutes, or they will become too dry and hard.

6. Remove the cookies from the oven, and let cool for 5-10 minutes on the baking sheets. Then transfer to wire racks to cool completely. Serve cookies

immediately, or keep them stored in an airtight container at room temperature or in the freezer.

Nutritional Data

Calories: 124

Total Fat: 9

Carbohydrates: 4

Fiber: 2

Protein: 5

•••

SNACK/DESSERT RECIPE: CHOCOLATE-DIPPED MACAROONS

Servings: 10 - Yield: 20 macaroons (Serving Size: 2 cookies) Total Time – Prep to Finish: 1 hour 35 minutes (inactive: 1 hour chill time)

Ingredients

- 8 large pasture-raised egg whites
- ½ tbsp. Stevia powder extract (or 9-12 Stevia packets)
- 4 c. unsweetened shredded coconut
- 4 tbsp. coconut flour
- 2 tsp. almond extract
- ¼ tsp. sea salt, or to taste
- 12-16oz. vegan semisweet or dark chocolate chips

Directions

1. Preheat oven to 325F. Line 2 baking sheets with parchment paper.

2. In a large mixing bowl, whisk the egg whites, Stevia, almond extract, and salt.

3. Then add in the coconut and flour, and mix until well incorporated.

4. Set in the refrigerator for 1 hour to harden.

5. Scoop the dough into 1-inch semi-rolled pieces, and lay the pieces on the parchment-lined baking sheet. Bake for 18-20 minutes or until the macaroons are lightly toasted and the bottom edges are golden brown. Remove from oven, and let cool completely.

6. Melt the chocolate chips in the microwave or double boiler. Dip the top of each macaroon in chocolate and place the dipped macaroons on a sheet of parchment or wax paper to set. Let the chocolate harden at room temperature or in the refrigerator. Once the chocolate is firm, serve and enjoy! Yield: 20 macaroons

Nutritional Data

Calories: 250
Total Fat: 16
Carbohydrates: 27
Fiber: 3
Protein: 4

●●●

CRISPY BUTTERSCOTCH COOKIES

*Cost Conscious Meal: Cookies make excellent budget-friendly treats since they usually use common ingredients found in most household pantries. One batch typically yields a large number of cookies, enabling you to freeze some and store some in airtight containers at room temperature for quick treats anytime!

Servings: 12 – Yield: 24 cookies (Serving Size: 2 cookies) Total Time – Prep to Finish: 25 minutes

Ingredients

- 2 c. almond flour
- ¼ c. coconut oil
- ¼ tbsp. Stevia extract powder (or ¼ tsp. liquid Stevia OR 5-6 Stevia packets)
- 1 tsp. agave nectar
- ½ tsp. butterscotch extract
- ¼ tsp. sea salt

Directions

1. Preheat oven to 350°F. Line a baking sheet with parchment paper.
2. In a medium mixing bowl, mix together the almond flour, coconut oil, Stevia, agave nectar, butterscotch extract, and sea salt until a nice dough forms.

3. Form 1-inch balls with the dough, and place the dough balls on the parchment-lined baking sheet. You should have enough dough to make 24 balls.

4. Flatten cookies gently by stamping with a fork. Once with the fork tines straight up and down and once side to side. You will make a cross shape with your fork.

5. Place in the preheated oven and bake 8 – 10 minutes or until lightly browned around the edges. Remove from oven, let cool for at least 5 minutes before serving.

Nutritional Data

Calories: 88
Total Fat: 9
Carbohydrates: 7
Fiber: 1
Protein: 1

●●●

ALMOND BUTTER "GRANOLA" BARS

Servings: 14 - Yield: 14 bars (Serving Size: 1 bar)
Total Time – Prep to Finish: 15 minutes

Ingredients

- 1½ c. almond butter

- 1½ c. white sesame seeds

- 2 tbsp. agave nectar

- ½ c. unsweetened flaked coconut

- ½ c. sunflower seeds OR pumpkin seeds
- ½ c. walnuts, chopped fine
- ½ c. pecans, chopped fine
- Stevia, to taste
- 2 tsp. cinnamon
- 1 tsp. vanilla extract
- 1/8 tsp. sea salt

Directions

1. Preheat oven to 350°F. In a large mixing bowl, combine the almond butter, agave nectar, Stevia, cinnamon, vanilla extract, and sea salt. Mix until well-blended.

2. Next, add to the mixing bowl the shredded coconut, sesame seeds, and sunflower seeds (or pumpkin seeds). Blend together thoroughly.

3. In a food processor, chop walnuts and pecans, and then transfer the chopped nuts to the peanut butter mixture. Blend well.

4. Press the mixture into a 9- x 11-inch baking dish, and bake for 9 to 11 minutes or until slightly browned.

5. Remove from heat, flip out onto a piece of parchment paper, and let cool completely before serving, storing, or freezing.

Nutritional Data

Calories: 247

Total Fat: 21

Carbohydrates: 8

Fiber: 2

Protein: 8

●●●

APPLE NACHOS WITH CHOCOLATE AND NUT TOPPINGS

Servings: 1 (Serving size: 1 apple wedged with toppings)
Total Time – Prep to Finish: 10 minutes

Ingredients

- 1 large Granny Smith green apple, cut into wedges
- 1 - 2 tbsp. (fresh lemon juice, more or less as needed just to splash the apple wedges
- ¼ - ½ c. almond butter
- ¼ c. vegan chocolate chips, divided (such as Enjoy Life)
- ¼ c. unsweetened shredded coconut
- 1-2 tbsp. almonds, sliced

Directions

1. First, slice the apple and place the wedges in a bowl. Squeeze the lemon juice over the bowl and toss to coat.

2. Arrange the apple wedges on a dessert plates.

3. Using a pastry/piping bag or a Ziploc bag, drizzle the almond butter over the apple wedges.

4. Finally, sprinkle the dish with ¼-½ c. shredded coconut, ¼- ½ - c. chocolate chips, and 1-2 tbsp. sliced almonds. Serve and enjoy!

Nutritional Data

Calories: 158
Total Fat: 12
Carbs: 13
Dietary Fiber: 2
Sugars: 5
Protein: 3

YOGURT VEGETABLE DIP

Ingredients

- 2 cups plain Greek or goat's milk yogurt
- 1 cup diced cucumber
- 2 tbsp finely chopped fresh dill
- 2 tbsp fresh lemon juice
- 2 cloves of minced garlic
- Salt and pepper to taste

Directions

- Combine yogurt, cucumber, garlic, lemon juice, and dill. Add salt and pepper to taste. Chill before serving.

●●●

GREEN SMOOTHIE

Ingredients

- 2 cups of kale, 1 head romaine lettuce, 2 cups spinach, or combination of the 3
- ½ cup coconut milk
- 1 scoop Vanilla or Chocolate Perfect Protein
- 2-3 tablespoons cocoa powder
- ½ avocado
- 1-2 cups of crushed ice (depending on desired consistency)
- Stevia to taste

Directions

1. Put the lettuce, kale, and/or spinach in the blender with avocado and the coconut milk.
2. Blend until greens are fully mixed.
3. Add ice, cocoa powder, and Perfect Protein and mix until well blended.

●●●

MIXED SWEET NUTS

Ingredients

- 5 cups of raw, whole almonds and/or pecans
- 1 Egg white
- 1 tbsp of water
- 1/2 cup Xylitol
- 1tbsp cinnamon

- Pinch of salt

Directions

1. Mix together.

2. Cook for 15 min at 350 degrees.

3. Stir and cook for another 10-15 min until browned.

●●●

CHOCOLATE MALTED SMOOTHIE

Ingredients

- 1 cup coconut milk
- 1-2 cups of ice (depending on desired thickness & consistency)
- ½ avocado (Makes it like a malt)
- 1 tablespoon of almond or peanut butter
- 2-3 tablespoons of unsweetened cocoa powder
- 1 scoop Chocolate Perfect Protein

Directions

- Mix ingredients in a blender until desired consistency.

●●●

SNACK/DESSERT RECIPE: CHOCOLATE CHIA PUDDING

Ingredients

- 1 can of organic coconut milk

- 4 tablespoons of chia seeds

- 1.5 scoops of ML Chocolate Perfect Protein (Can make it pack even more of a protein punch with a tablespoon of organic, unsweetened cocoa powder and Stevia to taste)

Directions

1. Mix ingredients together until it makes a smooth solution with no clumps.
2. Refrigerate until it hardens.

●●●

SNACK/DESSERT RECIPE: CHOCOLATE AVOCADO PUDDING (1 SERVING)

Ingredients

- 1 avocado, soft and ripe
- 1 teaspoon vanilla
- 1/4 cup cocoa powder
- Stevia to taste

- 6 tablespoons coconut milk (Or just water if cutting calories)
- ¼ cup of ice
- (Even better with a scoop of Perfect Protein)

Directions

1. Cut avocado in half, and remove pit. Scoop out flesh, and put in in the blender along with remaining ingredients.
2. Process until smooth, occasionally scraping down sides. Serve immediately, or refrigerate until ready to serve. Ice keeps it from getting hot in the blender, so you can eat it right away.

Nutrition data (per serving)

kCalories: 580
Fat: 47 (18 grams monounsaturated, 25 grams saturated, 4 grams polyunsaturated)
Carbohydrates: 29
Fiber: 16
Protein: 10

●●●

SNACK/DESSERT RECIPE: CHOCOLATE ALMOND-BUTTER FUDGE (8 SERVINGS)

Ingredients

- 1 cup dark chocolate chips (73% dark)

- 1 cup almond butter
- 2 tbsp Xylitol
- ½ tbsp vanilla extract
- ¼ tsp sea salt

Directions

- Melt chocolate in medium pot. Remove from heat, and stir in almond butter and Xylitol.
- Once incorporated, stir in vanilla and salt.
- Spread into a loaf pan, and refrigerate for at least 2 hours. Cut quickly into small squares, and store in fridge or freezer.

Note: if using unsweetened chocolate, use more Xylitol. If chocolate is less than 73% dark, eliminate Xylitol.

Nutrition data (per serving)

kCals: 350
Fat: 28 (16 grams monounsaturated, 7 grams saturated, 5 grams polyunsaturated)
Carbohydrates: 18
Fiber: 5
Protein: 6

●●●

SNACK/DESSERT RECIPE: COCONUT MACAROONS (12 MACAROONS)

Ingredients

- 1 cup organic raw almonds
- 2 cups unsweetened coconut flakes
- 1 scoop Maximized Living vanilla protein powder
- 3 Tbsp organic unsweetened cocoa
- Stevia or Xylitol to taste.
- 7 Tbsp warm (liquid) coconut oil
- 1 Tbsp flax seeds

Directions

1. In blender or food processor grind almonds, flax seeds, and sesame seeds. Blend in remaining ingredients.
2. Remove mixture, and place tablespoon-sized macaroons on a cookie sheet or shallow baking dish and chill.

Nutrition data (per macaroon)

kCals: 200
Fat: 17 (5 grams monounsaturated, 8 grams saturated, 2 grams polyunsaturated)
Carbohydrates: 6
Fiber: 3

ENDNOTES

Chapter 2

1. *Psychosomatic Medicine: Journal of Biobehavioral Medicine.* University of Waterloo, news release, Sept. 15, 2014.

2. Kaplan, J. T., Gimbel, S. I., & Harris, S. "Neural correlates of maintaining one's political beliefs in the face of counterevidence." *Scientific reports,* 6: article 39589.

3. Wansinski, B., & Sobal, J. (2007). "Mindless eating." *Environment and Behavior,* 39 (1): 106.

4. Henry, H. Y. (2010). "The sensorimotor striatum is necessary for serial order learning." *Journal of Neuroscience,* 30 (44): 14719-14723.

5. Wansinski, B., & Kim, J. "Bad popcorn in Big Buckets: Portion size can influence intake as much as taste." *Journal of Nutrition Education and Behavior,* 37 (5): 242-245.

6. Adams, K. F., et al. "Overweight, obesity, and mortality in a large prospective cohort of persons 50 to 71 years old." *New England Journal of Medicine,* 355 (2005-2006): 763-778.

7. Woods, S. C., & Ramsey, D. S. "Pavlovian influences over food and drug intake." *Behavioral Brain Research,* 110 (2000): 175-182.

8. Geier, A. B., Rozin, P., & Doros, G. "A new heuristic that helps explain the effect of portion size on food intake." *Psychological Science,* 17 (2006): 521-525.

9. Rogers, P. J., & Blundell, J. E. "Investigation of food selection and meal parameters during development of dietary induced obesity." *Appetite,* 1 (1980): 85-88.

10. Rolls, E. T. "Central nervous mechanisms related to feeding and appetite." *British Medical Bulletin,* 37 (1981): 131-134.

Chapter 3

1. Kruger, J., & David, D. "Unskilled and unaware of it: How difficulties in recognizing one's own incompetence lead to inflated self-assessments." *Journal of Personality and Social Psychology,* 77 (6) (1999): 1121-1134.

2. Ariely, D., & Wertenbroch, K. "Procrastination, deadlines, and performance: Self-control by precommitment." *Psychological Science* 13 (3) (2002): 219-224.

3. Nickerson, R. S. "Confirmation bias: A ubiquitous phenomenon in many guises." *Review of General Psychology* 2 (2) (1998): 175-220.

4. Abramson, L. Y., Seligman, M. E., & Teasdale, J. D. "Learned helplessness in humans: Critique and reformulation." *Journal of Abnormal Psychology,* 87 (1) (1978): 49-74.

5. Leach, J. "Cognitive paralysis in an emergency: The role of the supervisory attentional system." *Aviation, Space, and Environmental Medicine* 76 (2) (2005): 134-136.

Chapter 4

1. Fointiat, V., & Pelt, A. "Do I know what I'm doing? Cognitive dissonance and action identification theory." *Spanish Journal of Psychology*, 27 (2015): 18.

2. Robert Frost, "The Road Not Taken": http://www. bartleby.com/119/1.html.

3. Heubner, D. M., Neilands, T. B., Rebchook, G. M., & Kegeles, S. M. "Sorting through chickens and eggs; A longitudinal examination of the associations between attitudes, norms, and sexual risk behavior." *Health Psychology*, 30 (1) (2011): 110-118.

Chapter 5

1. L. E. Hebert, P. A. Scherr, J. L. Bienias, D. A. Bennett, D. A. Evan, "Alzheimer Disease in the U.S. Population: Prevalence Estimates Using the 2000 Census," *Archives of Neurology* 60, no. 8 (August 2003): 1119-1122.

2. Elizabeth Cohen, "CDC: Antidepressants Most Prescribed Drugs in U.S.," http://www.cnn.com/2007/ HEALTH/07/09/antidepressants/index.html (accessed December 9, 2010).

3. *U.S. Census Bureau Population Estimates* by Demographic Characteristics. Table 2: "Annual Estimates of the Population by Selected Age Groups and Sex for the United States: April 1, 2000 to July 1, 2004" (NC-EST2004-02). Source: Population Division, U.S. Census Bureau Release Date: June 9, 2005; http:// www.census.gov/popest/national/asrh/; http://www.

census.gov/popest/national/asrh/ (accessed December 9, 2010).

4. Ibid.

5. Ibid.

6. Ibid.

7. *Journal of the American Medical Association,* 295 (2006): 1549–1555.

8. Candis McLean, *The Report News Magazine,* January 22, 2005.

9. autismspeaks.org.

10. Ferrucci, L. & Alley, D. "Obesity, disability, and mortality." *Archives of Internal Medicine,* 167 (2007): 750-751.

11. "So Young and So Many Pills": The Wall Street Journal; Dec. 28, 2010; https://www.wsj.com/articles/SB100014 24052970203731004576046073896475588.

Chapter 6

1. Mischel, W. et al. (1989). "Delay of gratification in children." *Science,* 244 (4907): 933–938.

2. Metcalfe, J., & Mischel, W. "A hot/cool system analysis of delay of gratification: Dynamics of willpower." *Psychological Review,* 106 (1) (1999): 3–19.

3. Casey, B. J. et al. "Behavioral and neural correlates of delay of gratification 40 years later." *Proceedings*

of the National Academy of Sciences, 108 (36) (2011): 14998–15003.

4. Adams, K. F. et al. "Overweight, obesity, and mortality in a large prospective cohort of persons 50 to 71 years old." *New England Journal of Medicine,* 355 (2006): 763-778.

5. Taheri, S., Lin, L., Austin, D., Young, T., Mignot, E. "Short Sleep Duration Is Associated with Reduced Leptin, Elevated Ghrelin, and Increased Body Mass Index." *PLoS Med* 1 (3) (2004): e62. doi:10.1371/journal.pmed.0010062.

6. The National Weight Control Registry: http://nwcr.ws/.

7. Wing, R. R., & Phelan, S. "Long-term weight loss maintenance." *The American Journal of Clinical Nutrition,* 82 (1) (2005): 222S-225S.

8. Adriaanse, M. A. et al. "Planning what not to eat: Ironic effects of implementation intentions negating unhealthy habits." *European Journal of Social Psychology,* 40 (7) (2011): 1277-1293.